Vibrational Acupuncture

Vibrational Acupuncture

Integrating Tuning Forks with Needles

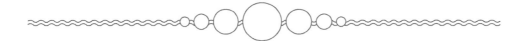

MARY ELIZABETH WAKEFIELD
and MICHELANGELO

Foreword by Donna Carey

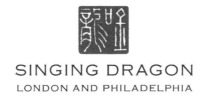

SINGING DRAGON

LONDON AND PHILADELPHIA

First published in 2020
by Singing Dragon
an imprint of Jessica Kingsley Publishers
73 Collier Street
London N1 9BE, UK
and
400 Market Street, Suite 400
Philadelphia, PA 19106, USA

www.singingdragon.com

Library of Congress Cataloging in Publication Data
A CIP catalog record for this book is available from the Library of Congress

British Library Cataloguing in Publication Data
A CIP catalogue record for this book is available from the British Library

ISBN 978 1 84819 343 7
eISBN 978 0 85701 299 9

Printed and bound in Great Britain by Ashford Colour Press Ltd.

Contents

Foreword

With the clear voices of master teachers, Mary Elizabeth Wakefield and MichelAngelo share their collective wisdom and years of experience to offer a beautiful synergy of sound-based therapeutics and acupuncture. From ancient China to ancient Greece, they trace the rich legacy of sound and music in the healing arts, while offering a modern, clearly articulated vision for contemporary and future medical practices, rooted in pioneering work in constitutional and facial acupuncture. The practical, immediately applicable techniques add credence to the efficacy of sound-based therapeutics, integrated with acupuncture, or as stand-alone treatments.

Whether you are an acupuncturist, an integrative medical practitioner, a student or practitioner of Acutonics® or this invaluable guide will deepen your understanding of acupuncture and Chinese medicine, ancient and modern practices. Even if you have been practicing for many years, you will find rich new information to aid in supporting your clients. Sound vibration, used with a depth of understanding and clear intention, has the power to impact all levels of our being, from the deep cellular level to the emotional, physical and spiritual.

When the initial vision for Acutonics® arose, in the early 1990s, the trend in acupuncture colleges was to become more Westernized. The spirit and deep lineage of the medicine were being lost. At the time, as a young acupuncturist, I envisioned a new type of school that would train practitioners in their sacred responsibility as physicians and remind them of the importance of cultivating both intuitive and scholarly knowledge, reclaiming the wisdom traditions of East and West. I was fortunate to have the support of a leading acupuncture college, where I served as Clinical Dean from 1995–2000 with responsibility for the creation of

14 community clinics. From the very beginning, I was driven to develop a therapy that was non-invasive and could be integrated into the practice of Chinese medicine. Our first Acutonics® classes were offered in 1998 through the college and the modality quickly became a favorite of patients and students. I understood at an intuitive level that the application of sound vibration, in particular the frequencies of the Earth, Moon, Sun and Planets, to meridians and acupoints would help to reconnect the individual with universal cycles that embrace mind, body and spirit as one, supporting patients through all phases of life.

I first met Mary Elizabeth and MichaelAngelo over the telephone in the winter of 2002—at that time the integration of sound-based therapeutics into the practice of acupuncture was still in its infancy. Our wide-ranging spirited phone conversations led them to drive nine hours from Tucson to Northern New Mexico, where together we welcomed in the New Year of 2003. This lively celebration was a time of sharing and deep conversation as Acutonics® Co-founder, Ellen Franklin, and I had truly found like-minded new friends who shared our vision yet brought their own unique insight. At our initial meeting we shared many ideas about sound-based therapeutics, gems, light and essential oils—things we envisioned as the future of medicine.

In March of 2003, Mary Elizabeth and MichelAngelo returned to Northern New Mexico to study Acutonics®. They continued their studies throughout 2003 and 2004. In 2004, Mary Elizabeth began collaborating with us on the development of gem tips for the Acutonics® tuning forks and MichelAngelo stepped in to assist in the teaching of our advanced classes. He went on to serve as an advisor on Astrological Medicine/ Musical Studies through 2013. He was also a contributor to our 2nd book, *Acutonics from Galaxies to Cells: Planetary Science, Harmony and Medicine*, published in 2010.

It is not often that you find genuine collaborators who are able to pursue their own unique path while also respecting and supporting the work of others. Ellen and I are both deeply grateful for this true and long-standing collaboration, and it was with genuine pleasure that we read an advance copy of *Vibrational Acupuncture*. Whether you are an experienced acupuncturist, or new to the field, or a practitioner of Acutonics®, you will find rich examples of the direct application of sound-based therapeutics to improve health and well-being. Additionally, for those seeking to more deeply understand Chinese medicine, which is at the root of Acutonics®, this book will take you on a step-by-step journey with clarity and rich practical applications, from constitutional work to a focus on internal and external beauty.

The synergies between Mary Elizabeth and MichelAngelo's unique vision and ours have been strong and powerful. This new book is a testament to their own unique voices and a welcome addition to the Acutonics® body of work.

From the great Western teachers, healers, and philosophers—Pythagoras, Plato, Asclepius, Chiron, Hygea, Ficino—to the great Chinese Eastern teachers, healers, and philosophers—The Yellow Emporer, Lao Tzu, Chung Tzu, Confucius, Pearl Mother of the West—the traditions of sound, light, essences, music, and poetry are embedded in the very fabric of this rich text. It is a sublime gift during these times of chaos and deep emotional, physical, psychic and environmental pain to find the clinical gems of practical applications to support people though the cycles of life.

To fellow pioneers, colleagues and friends, who have supported and been a part of the growth of Acutonics® around the globe, congratulations on this huge, rich and inspirational accomplishment.

Donna Carey, L.Ac.
Co-Founder, Acutonics Institute of Integrative Medicine, LLC
Llano, New Mexico

Acknowledgements

Cultivate the habit of being grateful for every good thing that comes to you, and to give thanks continuously. And because all things have contributed to your advancement, you should include all things in your gratitude.

Ralph Waldo Emerson

Writing this book has provided us, as partners of almost 27 years, with an experience that has been both enriching and compelling from a variety of perspectives. While our partnership has encompassed most aspects of our shared lives—musical, educational, and literary—it has now extended itself to the co-authorship of this groundbreaking book, *Vibrational Acupuncture: Integrating Tuning Forks with Needles.* Our educational outreach over the past 15 years as partners in *Chi-Akra Center for Ageless Aging* has provided us with a solid basis of dynamic collaboration and teaching experience, which has proven to be invaluable for this task. We feel that this book represents an authentic and original contribution to the field of complementary medicine.

Therefore, we would like to acknowledge ourselves, first, for the successful completion of a monumental effort. *Bravi!* Despite the stresses that inevitably accompany the gestation and eventual birthing of a book of this nature, we are still together! We hope that the teachings offered within will contribute to the development of a recognized and effective healing modality for professionals and laypeople alike.

We have both been professional opera singers who performed on the international level and are likewise Acutonics® practitioners. In the latter capacity, we are the co-creators of *Facial Soundscapes™*, a five-level certification program that utilizes the gamut of Acutonics® tuning forks.

Some of the discoveries that we made in the course of assembling and teaching these five seminars to practitioners from around the world have contributed, in a decisive way, to the techniques and information found in this book.

In addition to the shared operatic career, Mary Elizabeth Wakefield (MEW), L.Ac., M.S., M.M., is also a flutist, licensed acupuncturist, cranio-sacral and shiatsu therapist, internationally recognized teacher in the Chinese medicine field, and the author of a definitive work on facial acupuncture, *Constitutional Facial Acupuncture*[1] (and a German version published by Urban & Fischer). Mary Elizabeth has also contributed articles on facial acupuncture and related topics to a wide range of international acupuncture journals and spa periodicals.

MichelAngelo, M.F.A., C.T.M., is a published composer of classical art songs, pianist, medical astrologer, healer, diviner, and writer, who has had a number of articles published in international astrology journals and Chinese medicine magazines. He recently self-published an e-book of astrological essays, *Random Ramblings of an Astrological Autodidact*, on Amazon. For seven years, he served as Advisor, Astrological Medicine and Musical Studies to the Acutonics® Institute of Integrative Medicine, LLC, and was the principal creative partner of its co-founder Donna Carey, L.Ac. In this capacity, he also co-authored the advanced-level textbook *Acutonics from Galaxies to Cells: Planetary Science, Harmony and Medicine*.[2]

It should be noted that both of us, in separate ways, have come to the healing arts from the realm of the performing arts, and this blending of disciplines informs this book in ways that we think you will find quite unique.

However, you would not be holding this child of our efforts in your hands were it not for the influence of a number of wonderful people worldwide.

First of all, we'd like to acknowledge our senior commissioning editor for Singing Dragon UK, Claire Wilson, who, as her content strategist at Elsevier UK, was the principal "midwife" for MEW's book, *Constitutional Facial Acupuncture*—it was Claire who had the temerity to ask her if she'd like to write another book! It was also Claire who initially shepherded MEW through all the requisite steps for publishing a textbook with a major publisher, which were considerable. This is *our* "maiden" voyage into the wonderful world of publishing; consequently, this outing has seemed much less formidable, although it still required a sustained and concerted effort.

Claire also openly embraced, as did Jessica Kingsley, founder of Singing Dragon, the idea of a book that introduced an innovative synergy of these two modalities. Thank you, Claire, for your unflagging support and your ready availability and willingness to answer the slightest question on a timely basis. MEW also appreciates your sense of humor and your friendship, and MichelAngelo looks forward to meeting you in person in the not-so-distant future!

Many thanks to Maddie Budd, editorial assistant at Singing Dragon UK, for the help she provided with the editing of our manuscript. We'd also like to express our heartfelt admiration of the visionary Jessica Kingsley, who founded Singing Dragon in 2006 as a publishing house dedicated to books on the literature of healing—acupuncture, Chinese medicine, Daoism, Qi-gong, meditation, yoga therapy, massage, body work, Ayurvedic medicine, homeopathy, childbirth, children's books, etc.

It was at the end of a lengthy automotive pilgrimage all the way from Tucson, AZ, to the remote mountains of northern New Mexico that we first encountered the "tuning fork ladies," Donna Carey, L.Ac. and Ellen Franklin, Ph.D.; it is safe to say that, had we not made that exhausting trip, this book would never have been written!

Just prior to New Year's Eve, 2003, we arrived at their "Mothership" in the beautiful valley of Llano de San Juan. MEW was nursing a painful bladder infection that had worsened en route; after greeting us warmly, Donna immediately whisked her into the treatment room for a combined tuning fork/gong session—within 30 minutes, the bladder infection had passed, and MEW was able to join in the holiday celebrations!

This was the beginning of an intense and meaningful collaboration; Donna and Ellen invited us to participate in forthcoming Acutonics® seminars, and, as fate would have it, following the unanticipated and precipitate departure of Donna's then teaching partner, Marjorie De Muynck, MichelAngelo, with his specialized skills as astrologer and musician, was poised to step into the breach, and invited to become Donna's co-teacher and creative partner for a period of time.

While our relationship with Acutonics® has evolved and changed since then, we are grateful for their continuing friendship and their creation of a profound healing modality that emphasizes receptivity; you will be introduced to their remarkably effective planetary tuning forks later in this book.

We had no idea how fortunate we were to draw Annie McDonnell, L.Ac., sound practitioner, book editor at Hachette NYC, and founder of Joy Alchemy Acupuncture into our orbit earlier this year. Annie participated in three of our educational seminars, a certification series in *Constitutional Facial Acupuncture*™: *The New Protocols*, and two modules of our *Facial Soundscapes*™ training program, here in New York City.

Annie is accomplished in so many ways, and following our fortuitous meeting, was gracious enough to consent to pre-edit our manuscript. We warned her in advance that she would be working with authors with widely divergent writing styles and that we were counting on her to negotiate a middle ground, helping us to find the right manner in which to express our passionate convictions. With her understanding of Chinese medicine and sound therapy, and her skills as an editor, we were thrice blessed. Annie's contribution to this effort has been thoughtful, discerning, and highly professional. Thank you, Annie, for your wisdom and excellence.

We must also express our sincere gratitude to our gorgeous model, Lauren Cadillac, Registered Dietitian, C.P.T., and Certified Leap Therapist, one of MEW's acupuncture patients, and a colleague. She possesses a natural, unaffected beauty that mirrors her kindness and generosity of spirit. Despite her busy schedule, Lauren always made time for our various photo shoots. Thank you, Lauren, this book is enhanced by your luminous presence in it.

MichelAngelo was responsible for taking most of the photos, and all the formatting of the same for publication, the creation of the various graphics, and the input and formatting of the manuscript.

We'd also like to thank our colleagues and friends who have agreed to contribute something additional to the finished product:

- Donna Carey, L.Ac. co-founder of Acutonics®, for writing the foreword

- Susan Lange, O.M.D., L.Ac., Cynthia Reber Maman, B.A., Will Morris, Ph.D., D.A.O.M., M.S.Ed., L.Ac., *et al.*, for reviewing the finished work and sharing their impressions.

The depth of our gratitude to our dear friend Cynthia Reber Maman shows no bounds. After our departure from her home in Colorado, following a recent seminar in Denver, we discovered that our business laptop, containing the entirety of this manuscript, had inadvertently been left behind. We did not discover this fact until we had cleared security at Denver airport. Cynthia found the laptop hiding under a red blanket in her basement; perhaps it, too, didn't want to leave Colorado! This could have been disastrous, but she immediately FedExed it to us in New York overnight. This ensured that we would be able to complete our manuscript on schedule. Thank you, Cynthia—you are a true friend.

We are grateful for all our students worldwide—of the Wakefield Technique™ of facial acupuncture and *Facial Soundscapes*™—who have contributed to the expansion of our knowledge and experience. We especially wish to acknowledge those participants in our International GOLD STANDARD FACIAL ACUPUNCTURE® Certification Program, and our Certified Teachers, who are likewise its graduates. We are grateful for your enthusiasm for our teaching and your sharing of our philosophy.

Finally, we must humbly acknowledge the mysterious workings of Fate that unerringly steered both of us to a small town in Iowa some 27 years ago—we could not have anticipated that a seemingly chance encounter at a small opera festival in the Midwest would have such an impact upon our destinies and propel us to a newly shared life of abundant joy and rich creativity. Thank you, dear reader, for your investment in this latest creation of that mutual vision…

Mary Elizabeth Wakefield, L.Ac., M.S., M.M.
MichelAngelo, M.F.A., C.T.M.
Chi-Akra Center for Ageless Aging
New York, NY
www.facialacupuncture-wakefieldtechnique.com and chi.akra@gmail.com
Spring 2019
Year of the Golden Pig

Introduction

Yet everything that touches us, me and you,
takes us together like a violin's bow,
which draws one voice out of two separate strings.
Upon what instrument are we two spanned?
And what musician holds us in his hand?
Oh sweetest song.

Rainer Maria Rilke

What Is Vibration?

Each organ and function within the body creates a vibration which
helps it maintain its equilibrium. These vibrations allow the body
to cooperate with its self-healing.

Alfred Tomatis

The *Oxford English Dictionary* defines vibration as "an instance, or the state, of vibrating."[1] The word stems from the Latin verb *vibrare*: to vibrate, to move in small increments, to and fro. It is a state of resonating, as in the vibrato of a violin or an operatic voice.

It is also an act or condition of being vibrated in a single complete vibrating motion—a quiver or quickening of Qi (energy) when the soul enters the body of a child. Vibration is sensed or experienced directly and has a distinct emotional quality or atmosphere.

The Nature of Sound

Vibration has motion, therefore all life is in motion...behind the whole Creation, the whole of manifestation, if there is any subtle trace of life that can be found, it is motion, it is movement, it is vibration.

Hazrat Inayat Khan

Everything that moves—from the smallest molecule to the planets in their unceasing orbits to the vast galaxies pinwheeling throughout the unfathomable reaches of the universe—generates a vibration that we may consider to be sound, even if it may be beyond the capacity of our human ears to register.

The ear, a miraculous organ, can detect frequencies ranging from 20 to 20,000 cycles per second (hertz or Hz). In fact, the entirety of the human body responds to sound vibration, and we can "hear" by means of our skin and the 206 bones in an adult skeleton. Scientific studies have demonstrated that every cell in our bodies may be regarded as a little "ear." Other research has shown that sound can produce beneficial changes to the autoimmune, endocrine, and neuropeptide systems.[2]

When in a relaxed state, our body and brain waves vibrate at eight cycles per second, which entrains us to the basic electromagnetic field of the Earth.

Historically, more meditations and prayers have been sung, rather than spoken, in spiritual and religious practices worldwide. Research shows that the use of sound, chanting, and singing can support spiritual awareness and the health of the body (soma).

Creation Mythology

The knower of the mystery of sound knows the mystery of the whole universe.

Hazrat Inayat Khan

Ancient creation myths explain how humans were called into being with sound, song, and the spoken word.

- ⟐ "Let us make man in our own image, after our own likeness," God said in Genesis 1:26, and the Divine spoken word manifested creation, male and female, to inhabit Earth.

- ⟐ In Vedic texts, Prajapati, the Creator, hatched from a cosmic egg and created human beings and all of nature with the resonant sound of his voice. The Mayans were called into being by the miraculous incantation sounded by their Creator's voice.

Most indigenous American Indian tribes attribute sound and song to the beginning of creation.

- ⟐ In the Hopi tradition, Spider Woman breathed life into man/woman, nature, animals, and fish by singing the creation song.

- ⟐ Navajos believe that the sound of the wind created the first man and woman; this breath of life can be likened to the sound that sang life into humanity.

In Chinese medicine, wind relates to the Wood element and the Liver meridian, which mystically connects to the Hun or soul. When a child is born, it breathes in the song of life, and when death comes, this breath is given back to creation. The Hun-soul remains eternal.

The Australian Aborigines' creation myths are ancient and date back almost 200,000 years! Their Dreamtime song is both a physical and metaphysical sound.

According to the late Yehudi Menuhin, classical violinist, sound does predate speech. In fact, research notes that the early use of the voice to produce speech can be traced back only about 8000 years, while singing and chanting arose half a million years earlier.[3]

> Men sang out their feelings long before they were able to speak their thoughts. But of course we must not imagine that "singing" means exactly the same thing here as in a modern concert hall. When we say that speech originated in song, what we mean is merely that our comparatively monotonous spoken language and our highly developed vocal music are differentiations of primitive utterances, which had more in them of the latter than of the former.[4]

Steven Mithen, a professor of archaeology from the UK, in his book *The Singing Neanderthals*, has advanced a theory positing that human musical intelligence is not merely a by-product of our communicative capabilities with language. Mithen's somewhat revolutionary idea is that music and language have a mutual origin in a form of "holistic" communication among early hominids. The additional attributes of this rudimentary language are described as "manipulative," "multimodal," "musical," and "memetic." Mithen abbreviates this aggregate of characteristics as "HMMMM," reinforcing the notion that this is a language that takes musical tone, rather than linguistic content, as its point of departure. This proto-communication engages both hemispheres of the brain, and he believes that his "vocal" Neanderthals would have transmitted ideas in this manner.[5]

Communication of this nonverbal, but musical, type would not be necessarily limited in scope. We can cite several modern languages, including Chinese, in which a myriad of potential interpretations of a single syllable are possible due to tonal variation of the relevant vowel sound. Thus, Mithen's Stone Age singers may indeed have been able to convey messages of some complexity with their "humming," even without a sophisticated or extensive vocabulary.

Based upon other recent archaeological evidence, it is arguable that our musical ability was manifest long before we developed sophisticated verbal communication. One of the world's most ancient musical instruments, approximately 30,000–37,000 years old, was unearthed by a team of German archaeologists in the mountains near Ulm, Germany, in 2004. The 18.7-centimeter-long flute, carved from mammoth ivory, has three finger holes and would have been capable of playing relatively complex melodies, based on the pentatonic scale—a fitting instrument for a Paleolithic musical virtuoso.

Two other flutes made of swan bones were discovered at the site more than a decade prior to this latest find, and these three wind instruments vastly predate any other such musical artifacts. It is the extraordinary sophistication of the newly discovered instrument that distinguishes it from the others.[6]

Children express themselves with song—singing and humming—long before they speak. The corpus callosum, the tightly wound bundle of nerve tissue that connects the twin hemispheres of the brain, is not yet fully developed. Therefore, the nonverbal, nonlinear, mystical, and creative right brain is more active in children and in left-handed adults.

As a child, I remember making sounds and mimicking music and tones, long before I could verbalize what I was feeling or thinking. *In utero*, while swimming in the timeless amniotic sea, we are immersed in sound! The amniotic fluid is an optimal medium for the conduction of sound waves. In fact, the embryo begins to develop ears as early as three weeks into pregnancy, and can feel and hear the beating of its mother's heart *in utero*. Research shows that when an infant is exposed to a recording of a heartbeat of 72 beats per minute, they will relax. Babies also respond to the mother's voice within 72 hours after birth.

In my experience, babies also recognize the voice of the practitioner who cared for the mother during her pregnancy. I asked one of my pregnant patients if I could sound and sing into her belly when her baby became distressed. In this way, I created nonverbal sounds and songs that relaxed him, as the mother bonded with her baby.

Several months after his birth, she returned to my office for a visit to introduce her beautiful boy to me, not realizing that he already knew me! The minute I said his name, he voiced a loud joyful "Hah!" and reached his pudgy arms out to me, wanting to be held. The mother was surprised until I explained that her child undoubtedly recognized my voice from those early experiences of it while in the womb and had entrained with the sound of my voice.

Cosmic sound is the power that generates the rotative motion of every globular form of existence...a power that precipitates the Divine Will into material, objective manifestation.

Dane Rudhyar

Sufi mystics believe that the sound of the human voice, the tones emitted from the vocal cords, can attune us with the vibrational network of the cosmos, the Music of the Spheres, as originally postulated by the Greek proto-philosopher Pythagoras. As we have previously established, sound is vibration, and we have the capacity to perceive these vibrational energies not merely with our ears, but in every cell of our bodies.

Although the experience with my patient's baby is not, strictly speaking, entrainment in the conventional sense, the sound of my voice, informed by intention, established a sympathetic resonance, a vibrational rapport, between me and the unborn child.

The first scientist to formally document this phenomenon of entrainment was 17th-century mathematician and astronomer Christiaan Huygens, from the Netherlands. He observed that when two clocks hung side by side, their pendulums would, over time, synchronize their swings. The rhythmic vibration of one clock caused the second one, of a similar frequency, to vibrate in resonance with the first. The two clocks had similar vibrations and entrained (literally, got on the train together!), because they were fellow rhythmic travelers, communicating with each other in a vibrational dance!

Similar rhythmic synchronization occurs throughout the universe –involving molecules and atoms, in cycles of activity and rest, day and night, light and dark. The ancient Chinese understood this flux and flow, which is reflected in their Yin/Yang theory.

Human beings also rhythmically vibrate together; when our Qi has a similar frequency or affinity with another, then our senses and bodies can respond to sound waves generated by our own or another's voice.

The Sufi master and musician, Hazrat Inayat Khan, spoke about how our bodies are rhythmic—our pulse, heart, breath, and cranial rhythms all have their own beats! Our bodies resonate on a cellular level, especially with the sound of the human voice, whether heard *in utero*, in a face-to-face conversation, or on the telephone. The vibrations and unique inflections, and the particular timbre of the voice, are recognized as a unique auditory imprint by the ear, which possesses an uncanny accuracy in this regard.

What Is Music?

The world is sound. We find music everywhere: in planetary orbits, pulsars, genes, oxygen atoms, leaf forms, etc.

Joachim-Ernst Berendt

Music is organized sound; most cultures since the beginning of recorded time, and most likely in prehistoric eras as well, have used music therapeutically, to reduce stress, strain, and pain, promote relaxation, foster awareness, improve learning, clarify values, and balance, bolster, and enhance Qi.

When an organ or part of the body is healthy, it creates a natural resonant frequency in harmony with the rest of the body; when out of harmony, it is dis-eased, uncomfortable with itself, reflecting pathogenic imbalances, according to Traditional Chinese Medicine. The use of "correct" sound can balance and harmonize unhealthy harmonic patterns in our body/mind/spirit.

Many methods of sound healing are currently being employed by a wide range of practitioners worldwide; they include mantras, chants, and the playing of acoustic instruments—tuning forks, Tibetan and crystal bowls, gongs, tingshas, bells, chimes, etc. Most powerful of all is the concerted and directed use of the human voice, which is informed by the intention of the practitioner.

> The *bel canto* human voice is for sound what a laser is for light: The voice is an acoustical laser, generating the maximum density of electromagnetic singularities per unit action. It is this property which gives the *bel canto* voice its special penetrating characteristic, but also determines it as uniquely beautiful and uniquely musical.[7]

Keening

An excellent example of this cathartic use of the human voice is found in the practice of keening. Since the 17th century, Irish and Scottish women have wailed with grief over recently departed loved ones at a funeral. This lament is accompanied by rocking back and forth, kneeling, or clapping their hands loudly, as they give voice to their loss. Often a chorus of women will keen in unison, wailing up and down through the entirety of their vocal range, to produce a sound like the siren of a fire truck.[8]

Tingshas

Tingshas resemble two small handheld cymbals that are joined by a piece of leather. Each cymbal is different, and when they are struck together, they produce a rapid "beat" or frequency that can be heard or felt. In fact, the beats arise because the interval that the two cymbals engender when sounding simultaneously is more dissonant than harmonious; hence, the peaks of the sound waves occur in greater proximity to each other.

Research shows that these frequencies (extremely low frequency, or ELF) vibrate between four and eight cycles per second (Hz), and entrain the brain waves to their pitch. In Tibetan Buddhism, tingshas are sounded before and after meditation to promote mindfulness and to bring attention to the present moment. They are usually cast from bronze, copper, tin, zinc, and nickel.

In modern practice, tingshas can be used before a treatment to promote relaxation and, after the session, to gently rouse the patient from a meditative state or slumber. They can also be resonated for space clearing in your office or home or, when traveling, in your hotel room.

An ancient religious group called the Bon, who predated Tibetan Buddhism, employed tingshas for the purpose of expelling ghosts, which are called Gui in Chinese medicine.

Tibetan Singing Bowls

Ancient caravan routes transported goods, new ideas, and religions across Asia, and subsequently two distinct sects of Buddhism developed in Tibet—Lamaism, which is basically Buddhism with strong Bon influences, and the Bon religion itself, which reflects more the shamanic aspect of Buddhism.

Historically, singing bowls were used for shamanic purposes, such as exorcising demons, and therefore their utility was not openly acknowledged by Tibetan Buddhists. However, both schools of Buddhism featured sound as a vital aspect of their rituals and meditations. Many people have heard and experienced the healing power of the overtone chanting of the Tibetan monks in their monasteries.

However, in Nepal, metal singing bowls are reserved for eating and drinking only, and the Nepalese either deny or are ignorant of this additional dimension. While the origin of these instruments is shrouded in mystery, it is believed that monks, or traveling metalsmiths, created the original singing bowls from seven planetary metals, one for each of the seven traditional planets in the solar system:

- Sun: gold

- Moon: silver

- Mercury: mercury

- Venus: copper

- Mars: iron

- Jupiter: tin

- Saturn: lead.

Each of these planetary metals produces a unique tone, and synergizing them creates exceptional harmonics. While bowls of this type are still being produced in Asia and imported to the West, knowledge of the precise metallurgical techniques employed in the production of the original bowls has not survived. Each bowl has its own unique vibratory signature.

- Tibetan bowls are available in various sizes, and also emit different types of sounds.

- The precise timbre of each bowl is determined by the shape of the bowl, the metals used, and the thickness of the rim.

- Bowls are decorated with nature motifs—leaves, stones, flowers— or with inscriptions of the Nepalese or Tibetan language.

- Calendar bowls, which are extremely rare, are ornamented with either the lunar calendar or one that is based on Jupiter and have a particular astrological significance. The Jupiter calendar can be regarded as akin to the Chinese zodiac of 12 animals, because the orbital cycle of Jupiter is 12 years in duration.

Crystal Bowls

Crystal bowls are made from almost 100 percent crushed quartz that is heated to about 4000 degrees Fahrenheit in a centrifugal mold. Crystals are fossilized water that is formed when water combines with an element, like silica sand, under conditions of pressure.

The human body, although comprised of organic tissue, flesh, blood, and bone, is, nevertheless, infused with a lattice of nerve fibers, through which information travels by means of electrochemical signaling; in a similar fashion, the structural matrices of quartz and other crystals respond with piezoelectric effects to certain external stimuli and can be programmed to transmit desired thought forms. Therefore, working with crystals can beneficially affect our organs, meridians, tissues, and circulatory, endocrine, and metabolic systems. Crystal bowls are manufactured in varying sizes and emit different notes, along with the associated overtones.

Tibetan singing bowls are forged and then shaped manually; the Buddhist masters say that a prayer is intoned with every blow of the hammer, infusing them with a million prayers of pure intention. Crystal bowls are also transformative tools that can be utilized to effect change in one's life. Approaching these bowls with a similar reverence, pure intention, and awareness can mirror and heal the crystalline nature of our being.

Gongs

The first gongs were probably created in China, during the Bronze Age, some 5000 years ago. Later, countries such as Indonesia, Thailand, Vietnam, and the Philippines began utilizing gongs as communication devices, because their vibrations could be perceived over long distances; their use was similarly important in religious rituals.

Like Tibetan bowls, gongs were hammered and shaped out of various metals: brass, bronze, copper, nickel, tin, and zinc. In more recent years, with the advent of music therapy, healing sound has come to the fore to address issues of sound pollution and the growing lack of receptivity caused by the dominance of eye-centered technologies, such as smartphones, in particular.

Gong baths have become a popular way to tune, tone, balance, and heal body/mind/spirit; the gong represents a creative, vibrational process. When the gong is struck at its center a deep fundamental tone arises, which divides the gong into harmonic and nodal patterns. If it is struck elsewhere on its surface, a partial tone is emitted, and a portion of its overtones are heard. Paiste, the German manufacturers of symphonic gongs, have created superior-quality gongs, attuned to a range of frequencies, including planetary tones, for purposes of sound healing.

Bells

Historically, bells predate singing bowls. In 1978, 65 orchestral bells were excavated from an archaeological site in the Hubei Province in China, dating from the Warring States period (c. 475–221 BCE). These tuned bells, used in rituals and for ceremonies, each weighed over 100 pounds, and produced two different tones when struck. The Chinese clearly possessed a highly developed knowledge of acoustics to create these precision-tuned instruments.

Bells are cast from bronze, while singing bowls are usually hammered, not cast. Both have featured prominently in transformational rituals, originating with earlier shamanic practices and then again later in a wide range of spiritual observances. In Buddhist prayer services, the bell was struck as a call to prayer; it symbolizes the Buddha's voice and the harmony of the Yin (feminine) and Yang (masculine). Bells summon the spirit and divine presences and, like tingshas, serve to delineate the beginnings and endings of meditations.

Tuning Forks

A tuning fork is an acoustic resonator in the form of a two-pronged fork with a handle. The prongs (tines) are fashioned from a U-shaped bar of elastic metal. Steel (or customarily with tuning forks employed in vibrational healing, an amalgam of high-grade space-age metals) is used for this purpose. The length of the tines is instrumental in the production of a specific constant pitch when the fork is activated by striking it against a surface or with an object. The fork emits a pure musical tone and, depending upon the length and mass of the resonators (the tines), this frequency can be of quite long duration, making these instruments extremely effective in addressing disharmonies within the physical or energetic bodies. When a tuning fork is first set into vibration, we hear a fairly loud note, but this resonance dissipates rather quickly as the frequency of the vibrations is transmitted to the surrounding air.

The tuning fork was invented in 1711 by John Shore (d. 1752), the renowned musician, instrument maker, and trumpeter to the English Royal Court and a favorite of the expatriate German composer George Frideric Handel (1685–1759). The main reason for using the fork shape is that, unlike many other types of resonators, it produces a very pure tone, with most of the vibrational energy confined to the fundamental frequency, i.e., the pitch of the fork, and very little in the way of overtones.

Another singular advantage of the tuning fork configuration is that when it vibrates, the characteristic oscillation of the prongs causes the handle to move up and down. Consequently, there is a node, a point of no vibration, at the base of each prong. The motion of the handle is largely undetectable to the person resonating the instrument, which permits the fork to be held without damping the vibration. It also allows the handle to transmit the vibration to a resonator, which amplifies the sound of the fork or, conversely, for the frequency to be absorbed by the human body via acupuncture points, muscles, and bone structure. Medical doctors traditionally use tuning forks as a diagnostic aid to detect broken bones.

Sound and Sacred Geometry

Life in its manifestation is vibration...all things that we see or hear, that we perceive, vibrate...

Edgar Cayce

Research has proven that sound waves engender geometric shapes in various media. Ernst F. F. Chladni (1756–1827), considered the father of modern acoustics, a German physicist and amateur musician, demonstrated that the power of sound vibrations has an impact on matter. In his experiment, he spread fine grains of sand, or iron filings, on a metal plate and caused the plate to vibrate by drawing a violin bow across the edge to produce a tone. The harmonics intrinsic to the frequency of the violin tone were translated to the physical medium of the sand, producing geometric shapes as the particles rearranged themselves in accordance with the overtones of the instrument.

Vibration...is the one basic substance and energy of all matter.

David Tame

Later, another notable acoustic experiment was conducted by the Welsh singer Margaret Watts-Hughes (1842–1907), author of *Voice Figures* in which geometric patterns occurring in nature were produced by the vibrations and associated overtones of the human voice. Ms. Watts-Hughes sang into an instrument called an eidophone, which consisted of a tube, a receiver, and a flexible membrane. As she sang through a musical scale, she observed that definite, recognizable forms appeared.

Her experiments prove that:

- sound waves produce shapes when passed through a physical medium, such as sand or a liquid, and engender characteristic patterns related to the frequencies employed

- to produce a particular form, you must sing a specific note or pitch

- specific frequencies give rise to distinct and individual patterns.

In the 1960s, Swiss-born Dr. Hans Jenny (1904–1972), who coined the term "cymatics"—a name that is derived from a Greek word meaning "wave"—devoted himself to the study of cycles. He adapted the Chladni plate, replacing it with a circular disk, which he stimulated with a piezoelectric crystal in the center of its base, using different frequencies to produce geometric shapes.

The vibrational mode of the physical body is a reflection of the dominant frequency at which it resonates.

Richard Gerber

The late British osteopath, Dr. Peter Guy Manners, later adapted Jenny's cymatics and applied the theory for use in the healing professions. Cymatics therapy uses a toning device to transmit the signature vibrations of healthy organs and tissues into diseased areas of the body. The dysfunctional body structure is reharmonized through the introduction of a vibrational signature that is associated with its naturally healthy state; in effect, the tissue is reprogrammed. Malfunctioning organic "software" is overwritten with the original energetic matrix, which returns it to optimal functioning.

All of these modalities create healthy sacred space and facilitate greater focus, magnifying the intensity of the practitioner's intention.

Music and Chinese Medicine

In ancient China, music was believed to be instrumental to the accomplishment of a variety of objectives: to treat the health and well-being of the body and psyche, to ensure conformity with established moral codes, and to address potential disharmony within the state. Paralleling a similar philosophy established in the 6th century BCE in Greece by Pythagoras and his successors, music also provided a means whereby human beings could achieve harmony with the cosmos, the abode of divinity:

> When one considers the relationship between music and the cosmos, Pythagoras and his followers immediately come to mind... It is not known whether the early Chinese...were influenced by Pythagoras' theories on the connection between numerical patterns and music... But, the possibility that the Greeks somehow influenced the Chinese on this matter, or vice versa, cannot be ruled out.[9]

The concerted use of music in this manner had an essentially practical and therapeutic goal, that of achieving balance and promoting increased longevity.

The history of music as medicine in China dates back to the Warring States period. Negative music was categorized as "excessive" in nature, and positive was judged accordingly by its moral nature and focus on properly balanced sounds.

As a therapeutic tool with both physiological and psychological applications, music was considered an important tonic for increasing the quality of life and life span, in both the individual and the state. In other words, music, in Chinese medicine terms, warded off physical and emotional pathogens.

According to the ancient Chinese, balanced music reflected the harmonious totality of existence—that of body and mind, society, the environment, and the cosmos. Different styles of music also indicated the ease or dis-ease of the heart-mind connection in a person:

> If there is too much [of any of the Six Illnesses], then disaster strikes: excessive Yin corresponds to illnesses of cold, excessive Yang, to illnesses of heat; excessive wind to illnesses of the extremities; excessive rain, to the illnesses of the gut; obsessive obscurity, to illnesses that entail confusion; and excessive brightness to illnesses of the heart-mind.[10]

The Chinese believed that the entirety of creation was informed by a network of essential correspondences, and they observed these Five Elements reflected in nature, humanity, sound, and the heavens. It is true, however, that the Wu Xing, customarily translated as Five Elements, does not refer to elements, *per se*, but rather five phases, or states of being, which are made to correspond with the seasons of the year.

In ancient Greece, the four root substances, first postulated by Empedocles,[11] consisting of earth, water, air, and fire, were thought to explain the nature and complexity of all creation in terms of simpler structural constituents. It was Plato who, in his dialogue *Timaeus*, first referred to these building blocks of matter as elements. His pupil Aristotle later contributed a fifth element, aether, as the *quintessence*. His reasoning was that whereas fire, earth, air, and water were earthly and corruptible, subject to change, they must, of necessity, be confined to what he described as the "sub-lunar" realm of imperfection. However, because the heavens were perceived to be eternal and incorruptible, the fixed stars and constellations could not possibly be composed of the four earthly elements but must embody a different, unchangeable, heavenly substance. These five elements are sometimes associated with the five Platonic solids, which 17th-century pioneering astronomer Johannes Kepler later attempted to correspond to the orbits of the Five Element planets—Mercury, Venus, Mars, Jupiter, and Saturn. We should note, however, that, in general, Western esoteric philosophy and disciplines, including astrology and alchemy, are centered on the original four elements.

In Chinese medicine, the Five Elements correspond directly with the five seasons, the five tastes, the five colors of the organ systems, the five planets, the five tones and modes… If any of these correspondences becomes excess or out of balance, they could contribute to an onset of one of the Six Illnesses and accompanying heart-mind imbalances.

Table 1.1 Five Element correspondence chart with musical tones and planets[12]

Element	Season	Organ	Taste	Color	Chinese tone	Planet	Western tone (approximate)
Wood	Spring	Liv/GB	Sour	Green	Chiao	Jupiter	A
Fire	Summer	Ht/SI; PC/TH	Bitter	Red	Chi	Mars	C
Earth	Intercalary period*	Sp/St	Sweet	Yellow	Kung	Saturn	F
Metal	Autumn	Lu/LI	Pungent	White	Shang	Venus	G
Water	Winter	Kid/Bl	Salty	Blue/black	Yu	Mercury	D

* The 18 days between summer and autumn (the "center").

The ancient sages and enlightened beings understood the fluctuation of the patterns of nature's Qi Yuan—the rhythm of Qi—as peaceful songs. The peaceful song, or harmonious sound, was a way to represent the human being living in harmony with nature, and served as a seasonal guide to this pursuit. This ultimate goal has been named TianRenHeYi, meaning the union between human being and nature, since at least the Warring States period (circa 475–221 BCE).[13]

Therefore, exposure to balanced music, "peaceful songs," was essential for humans to live in harmony with nature and the cosmos. This mirrors the Taoist philosophy of the Three Treasures—Heaven, Humanity, and Earth. The Three Treasures refer to those intrinsic and united forces that embody Heaven (Shen), Earth (Jing), and Humanity (Qi). Earth relates to inherited essence or genetics, Humanity to Qi or energy, and Heaven to spirit—radiating compassion from our hearts.

The Taoist goal was to nurture, enhance, and unify the Three Treasures by refining Jing into Qi, Qi into Shen, and Shen into openness, to become one with the Tao. When Jing, Qi, and Shen are in harmony, and informed by breath, meditation, balanced music, and disciplined exercise, it is possible to achieve immortality or, at least, a long, healthy life!

Ancient cultures were generally in agreement that there is a fundamental relationship between the type of music one experiences on a daily basis and health. According to the Chinese, a state of optimum health can be achieved by an immersion in music that promotes harmony with the order of Heaven. They also believed that "indulgences" of any kind—food, sex, alcohol, or sensual music—could contribute to illness, disturb the spirit, and thereby damage the heart-mind connection. Certain musical styles could lead to excess and imbalance, and different parts of the body were linked to these disharmonies, for example, arms, hands, legs, feet, and the sexual organs, which led to sexual desires and inappropriate touching of the body. Balanced music focused on meditation, intention, and harmonious emotions.

Xunzi, born in the Zhao Dynasty (c. 300 BCE), and one of the three preeminent Confucian philosophers of the classical period in China, emphasized the beneficial effects upon centrality, harmony, and the balance of music on individual physiology and moral psychology:

> Thus, when music is performed, then one's intent is pure, when ritual is cultivated, one's conduct is complete. One's ears and eyes are perspicacious and clear; one's blood and Qi are harmonized and balanced.[14]

This description of music and its effects on physiology is reminiscent of the reported clarity and balance a patient experiences when serotonin production is stimulated, and the neurotransmitter is released by the needling or vibrational stimulation of the appropriate acupuncture or acu-sound points in a treatment.

Xunzi also emphasized the medical, moral, and spiritual effects of music on the community and state. Once again, a distinction was made between excessive, ignoble, seductive sounds and balanced, noble, appropriate sounds.

Peaceful, orderly music gave each individual in the community and state a sense of well-being, similar to that invoked by a meditation, and chaotic, unbalanced music stimulated desire solely for fulfillment of the senses. Music and moderation were achieved through musical ceremonies and rites. In Chinese philosophy, moral integrity kept the body free from pathogens and disease.

Ritual was a stabilizing influence for the people, providing them with appropriate balance, clarity, and order. For example, Confucius did not sing on the days that he had wept, in accordance with the Chinese belief that this would have exhausted his emotions, confused his psyche, and invited the possibility of illness and even death.

The Huang Kung: The Yellow Bell

The origins of Chinese musical practices can be traced back to 2700 BCE, when they were established by Ling-Lun at the court of the legendary Yellow Emperor, Huang-Ti.[15] The ancient Chinese consciously sought to align the quotidian activities of their existence, especially their music, with cosmic principles, seeking to maintain ideal proportions that would facilitate a vital connection to Tian/Heaven. This philosophy is akin to that espoused by the Pythagoreans, and it was Pythagoras who, according to his biographers, first formulated a musical scale based upon planetary tones.

In order to standardize musical practice, the ancient Chinese created a unique system, using a foundation tone of absolute pitch, which represented a cosmic sound, the Huang Kung. The tone of this Yellow Bell was referred to as the Kung, and it was believed to be the direct manifestation of the divine will, i.e., that of the emperor himself.

The instrument used to produce this celestial frequency was a precisely tuned bamboo pipe, manufactured to precise and exacting standards. According to imperial law, the length of this bamboo resonator became a standard Chinese measurement, and its capacity to hold a specific number of grains of rice was likewise strictly regulated.

Given the paramount importance of this tonal benchmark, it is perhaps not surprising that the Imperial Office of Music was likewise responsible for the maintenance of all standard weights and measurements. An ancient text, *The Memorial of Music*, contains a warning relating to the detection of a discrepancy in the pitch of the Kung tone: "If the Kung is disturbed, then there is disorganization (in the Kingdom), and the Princes (in the Provinces) are arrogant."[16] Each province of the empire had in its possession a similar bamboo pipe, which was originally tuned to that in the imperial palace. In order to ensure that the Kung tone remained pure, the emperor would, at regular intervals, dispatch the Minister of Music to every province in the kingdom to check the local versions of the Yellow Bell for any deviations from the imperial standard.

It should be noted that the emperor did *not* send his generals; based upon the minister's assessment of the conformity, or lack thereof, in the frequency of the regional instruments, the emperor would then have certain knowledge that, for example, funds had been embezzled from the imperial treasury or that the military or the regional princes were thinking of rebelling and conspiring to attack the Imperial City.

Thus, this imperially sanctioned standard of harmony, the Huang Kung, was employed in a practical way to maintain peace and tranquility throughout the kingdom. It is astonishing to contemplate the otherworldliness of a civilization organized along such lines, one in which a harmony of intention would serve as the unifying strand of an entire culture.

> To embody the *Logos* was not believed to be the calling of only one person... All beings were its manifestation: all could aspire to that purity and illumination of consciousness whereby they became the perfect,

undistorted presence of the Word. And thus, the very *purpose* of Chinese music was towards this end...the raising and purifying of all.[17]

Researchers have determined that the pitch of the Kung tone was approximately an F, in Western tunings. However, the Kung tone varied periodically for a variety of reasons.

- ⬥ As astrological configurations changed, so did the universal harmonies.

- ⬥ Progression from one zodiacal month to another indicated the necessity for a modulation in musical standards.

- ⬥ The emperor of each new dynasty saw fit to establish their own basis for the Huang Kung, and thus a new Kung tone became the embodiment of heavenly harmony.

- ⬥ In modifying the Kung for these various reasons, rigidity was thereby avoided, and this permitted the Chinese people as a whole to more readily embrace change.

The Last Dynasty of China, the Qing (1644–1912 CE) ——

Upon his accession to the throne, the last emperor of China, Puyi, determined that the pitch of the Kung should be modified to the note D. One wonders whether the collapse of the millennia-old Chinese Empire and the traditions of Chinese culture can be attributed to mismanagement of this crucial element.

Prior to the Qing Dynasty, Roman Catholic missionaries had visited China and had brought their religious music with them, and, over time, it was only natural that educated Chinese people would also become interested in Western secular music. It is further documented that, for the very first time, the emperor permitted Western classical music to be performed in his court.

As professional opera singers and musicians, we have a great reverence for the esthetically beautiful and expressive compositions that are the legacy of the Western classical music tradition. However, as it evolved from the earliest forms, based on Greek prototypes, Western music became less than exclusively sacred in its essence. In the Renaissance and thereafter, it suffered an increasing alienation from those philosophical principles of cosmic tuning first established in Greece by Pythagoras and his descendants. By the time that the Chinese would have been exposed to it in the early 20th century, it was largely a secular phenomenon, which, despite its artistic appeal, would have been negative in its impact upon the populace.

The Loss of Heavenly Connection and the Demise of the Chinese Empire

With the introduction of these exotic foreign harmonies, music, which had also represented a moral and spiritual compass for the Chinese, was irretrievably tainted. Perhaps the hospitality of the emperor was the beginning of the end. No matter how esthetically pleasing this new music was, it did not adhere to the principles that were the cornerstone of Chinese musical philosophy.

With the blessing of the emperor, Western musical instruments were introduced, and professors of European music were accepted at his court. These emissaries of the West instructed the Chinese how to perform classical music, indoctrinating them in a tonal system that was diametrically opposed to that of their native culture.

A further corrupting influence was the subsequent arrival of Western popular music—jazz bands, blues singers, etc.—who found ready audiences in sophisticated metropolises like Shanghai and Hong Kong. Too late, the emperor realized the fatal error he had made in permitting the standards of music to deteriorate, and, although he tried to reinstitute the imperial musical paradigm, his efforts for musical reform went unheeded, and his voice fell on deaf ears. With his forced abdication in the wake of the Xinhai Revolution in 1912, 5000 years of Chinese imperial continuity came to an abrupt end.

Chapter Summaries

In the following chapters, we will progressively outline our philosophy and present unique treatment protocols for *Vibrational Acupuncture: Integrating Tuning Forks with Needles.* To greater facilitate your learning of this material, you will find diagrams, drawings, treatment photographs, and charts to clarify the details of the protocols and help you to successfully implement them in your practice, or for self-treatment.

Chapter 1, An Overview of Quantum Music Theory: The reader is provided with useful and necessary information concerning the musical component of healing sound treatments, including Pythagorean number theory, the world of number and musical tone, the archetypal significance and healing applications of musical intervals and overtones, and the conversion of planetary movement into sound.

Relevant anecdotes are included to illustrate this material. The planetary myth, archetype, and symbolism of the Acutonics Ohm®/ Earth tuning forks used in Vibrational Acupuncture™ treatments will be introduced.

Chapter 2, Practical Discernment: Tuning Forks and/or Needles?: This chapter provides practical information required for Vibrational Acupuncture™ treatments:

◈ benefits and contraindications for acupuncture and tuning fork usage

◈ discernment, knowledge, and awareness of when to integrate these two modalities

◈ supplies, treatment length and timeline, etc.

Chapter 3, The Eight Extraordinary Meridians and Our Genetic Imprint: The Eight Extraordinary meridians embody our prenatal Qi—the Jing level of treatment. Even though much has been written in recent years on these meridians by experts within the Chinese medicine community, there are, in our experience, no protocols that take into account the integration of tuning forks with acupuncture needles on the master/ couple points of these meridians. This chapter includes:

◈ "Fascia Talk": palpation of the fascia to determine which master/ couple points to use in a given treatment

◈ information on the psychospiritual aspects of these meridians, not found in customary sources; this is in addition to the physical aspects

◈ specific treatment protocols utilizing sacred geometry and the lemniscate, the planetary glyph for Earth, and Sound Tube.

Chapter 4, Anti-Exhaustion Treatments: Anchoring the Ying: Ying, postnatal Qi, supports lifestyle choices—a person's diet, exercise regimen, thoughts, emotions, etc. Treatments for this level target the root cause of physical and psychospiritual fatigue, i.e., noise and air pollution. Source Luo points for treating anxiety, anger, sadness, depression, and other imbalances are introduced. Also included are specific protocols for integrating tuning forks with acupuncture needling—the Twister, the "V" Vortex, and the Three Treasures treatment are discussed.

Chapter 5, Harmonizing the Wei: This chapter includes:

- definitions of motor and trigger points

- how and when they are used to harmonize the Wei Qi

- treatments using trigger/motor point protocols for specific syndromes, i.e., temporomandibular joint dysfunction (TMJ)

- palpation techniques and discernment of which modality is appropriate.

Chapter 6, Facial Acu-Sound Protocols: The reader will be introduced to two facial acu-sound protocols.

1. A basic facial balancing treatment using two Acutonics Ohm® tuning forks in tandem on the face. Specialized techniques for this protocol include:

   - activating the tuning forks

   - holding

   - gliding

   - sliding

   - rolling.

2. Troubleshooting: "Turkey wattles." The platysma muscle, an imbalance of which is associated with the appearance of a saggy, drooping neck, is treated using motor points, either with needles, tuning forks, or a synergy of both modalities. Diagrams will illustrate each step of the process.

Chapter 7, Vibrational Hara: The Five Element Japanese hara, or abdominal, treatment has been used for centuries to maintain health and well-being. Palpation techniques and discernment concerning which treatment to employ will be discussed in depth. Additionally, the reader will be provided with an overview of the Five Elements, as they pertain to sound, receptivity, and listening.

Chapter 8, Solo Sound Therapy Treatments: This chapter is written with an "ear" to the treatment of super-sensitive, needle-phobic patients and also for non-acupuncturists who may wish to take advantage of these non-needle protocols. All the acu-sound treatments in this book are very effective when performed with tuning forks alone.

The authors recommend three specialized treatments—the Grounding Protocol: A Vibratory Ritual of Earthing, the Sacred Mudra Ritual: Lacing the Three Jiaos, and a Corpus Callosum Vibrational Balancing treatment—for balancing the twin hemispheres of the brain. Photographs and charts are included.

Chapter 9, Vibrational Topical and Internal Treatments: A complete topical protocol using natural and organic products to enhance the efficacy of the treatments is included in this chapter. Readers will be introduced to the use of the following products from our herbal company, Muse L'Herbal USA:

 ⚜ The QuintEssentials™ 5 Element Planetary Gem Elixirs

 ⚜ VibRadiance™ 5 Element Planetary Essential Oils, infused with gem essence

 ⚜ *Crème Vitale ESP Rose*, an organic Bulgarian rose moisturizing cream

 ⚜ three organic essential oil hydrosols (Bulgarian rose, lavender, and neroli).

Chapter 10, A Personal Note from the Authors: Additional guidelines and personal recommendations, drawn from the authors' personal and professional experience.

Chapter 1

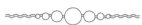

An Overview of Quantum Music Theory

Music, in its purest form, is an art which occurs in a specific location and time; musical tone, once emitted by any resonator, and propagated upon invisible, intangible waves that permeate the ambience of the performing space, imbues its resonance, as an expression of life force, of spirit soul, to every molecule of the atmosphere contained therein. Given voice to by a singer, or evoked by the appropriate actions of an instrumentalist, such sounds are ineffable, and only the semblance of them may perhaps be captured by even the most sophisticated recording equipment. This is a participatory paradigm, one in which both performer and listener are yoked in an intimate bond of intention and attention.

MichelAngelo

The Nature of Harmony

To the trained or instinctive musician, the principles of harmony are self-evident, and the structural constituents of music comprise a language that is readily comprehensible. However, for the individual for whom musical expression and knowledge is perhaps not second nature, the challenge of understanding the seemingly arcane principles of its organization may be somewhat more formidable.

We might best proceed by stating, at the outset, that the recognizable musical artefacts of our Western culture—vocal and instrumental, ranging from individual songs, both popular and classical, to the complex polyphonic structures of symphonies and operas, and everything between—are the result of individual creativity, unfettered, to a certain extent, by theoretical considerations. Yet, all great composers develop their individual musical style first by building upon the edifice of what has come before and what they have absorbed of the theory of composition from their studies and teachers. Music theory is, therefore, derivative in nature, with its precepts being extrapolated from the works of the authentic creatives, the composers. However, it does, as well, have its philosophical antecedents in the ancient world.

An Atomic Model

It may be helpful at this point to recognize that the smallest component of musical harmony is, in fact, a single tone, and make a comparison to a similarly minute constituent of physical matter. A musical tone can be likened to a single atom, in that it can be regarded as a self-contained cosmos, sublime in its simplicity. We are all familiar with the configuration of a typical atom; at its center is the nucleus, containing a definite number of protons and neutrons, analogous to the Sun at the heart of the solar system, surrounded by electrons moving in fixed orbits or shells. The acoustic "architecture" of an individual note can be likened to this and may additionally be construed as encoding the fundamental principles of harmonic structure, which are the expression of what we could certainly term natural "laws" of vibration.

What do we mean by this? In other words, a single tone manifests within its vibration certain indisputable symmetries. When the note low C (the note at the far left in Figure 1.1) is sounded on a Steinway grand piano, the other 15 tones (along with others) in this diagram arise, more or less simultaneously.

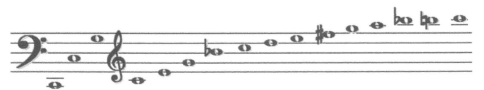

Figure 1.1 *The first 16 overtones of low C*

Why does this occur? For any given vibratory medium, for example a string, a length of hollow tube, the vibratory surface of the human vocal cords, etc., the longer the medium, the deeper the sound, i.e., the longer the wavelength of the vibration (the converse is also true). This is the reason that the bass notes on the piano sound "lower"—it is because they are generated by longer strings; men's voices have lower resonances than women's because they have larger larynxes that accommodate vocal cords of greater length.

We must bear in mind that the entire vibratory entity, whatever its nature, is a potential resonator; musical tone may ensue when any portion of it is sounded. This is the idea behind the monochord, a rudimentary instrument reportedly invented by Pythagoras, in which a single string is stretched over a board that has a moveable bridge; by varying the length of the vibrating string in moving the bridge, different frequencies will be produced. Each of these new sounds has a proportional relationship in numeric value to the fundamental tone; for example, if the bridge is moved to the halfway point along the string, the subsequent frequency heard will be precisely twice that, in hertz, of the base tone. This 2:1 ratio of string length and pitch may be regarded as a vibratory constant, expressed in musical terms as an *octave*. The octave is an essential organizing principle of vibration, whether it be that of sound or light.

To return to our Steinway grand piano, a more complex device for the production of sound, when the set of strings that are responsible for generating our low C are activated by depressing the key in the appropriate location on the piano keyboard, subsidiary vibrations, corresponding to the overtones of that particular frequency, likewise resound. As a general rule, most people cannot detect more than one or two of these evanescent additional vibrations, but, nevertheless, they do exist, and make their presence felt in the acoustic space and the character, or timbre, of the sound itself.

We might view this ensuing concatenation of overtones—or partials, because they represent, in this instance, parts of the vibrating strings, i.e., proportions thereof—from a different perspective. We have previously arrayed them in a linear fashion; in Figure 1.2 you will see them in a vertical alignment, resonating in what we could call a polychord. As a general rule, in the Western world we tend to think of musical harmony as relating to the vertical coincidence of tones. A chord is nothing more than three or more tones resounding simultaneously. One can easily play such a three-note chord on the piano, or strum it on the guitar.

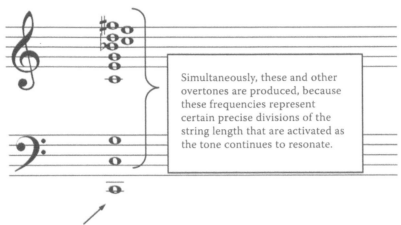

Simultaneously, these and other overtones are produced, because these frequencies represent certain precise divisions of the string length that are activated as the tone continues to resonate.

The vibrating string produces this tone, which is what the ear hears.

Figure 1.2 *Overtones of low C in a vertical array*

In keeping with our atomic metaphor, we might regard these ancillary tones, the overtones, of our bass note, C, illustrated above, as "haloing" the original pitch, almost like electrons, which, in their energetic shells, orbit the nucleus of the atom. While the atomic number, and essential identity, of any element is defined by the arrangement of protons and neutrons within the nuclear structure, it is the disposition of its electrons that determines its essential behavior and its capacity to become involved in chemical reactions.

The Importance of Overtones

In the same manner, without this gossamer adornment of its overtones, the sound of the fundamental tone, indeed the vast majority of musical frequencies, would seem bereft, even naked, more akin to that produced by some kind of electronic device than, in this instance, a Steinway piano.[1] It would lose much of its character and beauty to our ears.

Like electrons dancing around the atom's core, whose hierarchical arrangement in their successive energy shells obeys strict mathematical conventions,[2] each of these musical overtones comes into being as a vibratory multiple of the fundamental tone, as illustrated in Figure 1.3.

At the root, as we can observe in Figure 1.3, overtones are related to archetypes of number, and within their mathematically precise proportions they replicate the recognizable intervals of musical structure, which are defined by numerical ratios of 2:1, 3:2, 4:3, etc. Therefore, despite our modern Western notions of it, "harmony" is an intrinsic attribute of *all* musical sounds, because each tone is a self-contained universe of harmonic potential, expressed through its overtones. From this perspective, musical intervals represent the unfolding of that latent vibratory matrix into space and time: "A sound wave…is an electromagnetic process involving the rapid assembly and disassembly of geometrical configurations of molecules. In modern physics, this kind of self-organizing process is known as a 'soliton.'"[3]

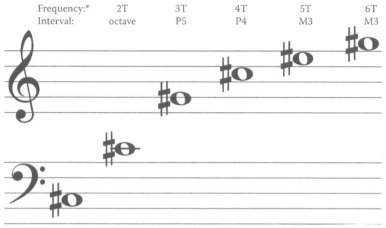

* If the frequency of the fundamental or tonic tone (T) is 110 Hz, the first overtone occurs at 220 Hz, the second at 330 Hz, etc.

Figure 1.3 *Overtones arise as precise multiples of the fundamental tone*

The regular ratios of musical intervals can be similarly extrapolated from a geometric figure known as the *tetraktys*, a Pythagorean symbolic construct that might be considered the cornerstone of his philosophy. But, who was Pythagoras, and what is the connection between Pythagorean number theory and music?

The First Philosopher

It can probably be argued that the study of music in the Western world begins and ends with this man, who, according to legend, coined the world "philosophy," i.e., love of knowledge:

> Greece of the 6th century BC evokes the image of an orchestra expectantly tuning up, each player absorbed in his own instrument only, deaf to the caterwaulings of the others. Then there is a dramatic

silence, the conductor enters the stage, raps three times with his baton, and harmony emerges from the chaos. The conductor is Pythagoras of Samos, whose influence on the ideas, and thereby, on the destiny, of the human race was probably greater than any single man before or after him.[4]

Pythagoras, born on the island of Samos in the Aegean Sea near the coast of Asia Minor, was the son of a gem engraver and silversmith named Mnesarchus. It is reasonably certain that he was a pupil of Anaximander, an Ionian philosopher and atheist, but also of Pherekydes, a mystic who taught the transmigration of souls. He must have travelled extensively in Asia Minor and Egypt, as many educated citizens of the Greek isles were wont to do, and it is said that he was charged with diplomatic missions by Polycrates, the enterprising autocrat of Samos.

All the ancient biographers agree that Pythagoras studied geometry in Egypt, where he was the first foreigner to be initiated into the Egyptian mysteries. In Phoenicia, he learned about "numbers and proportions," and in Chaldea (ancient Babylon and Sumeria), he received instruction in astronomy from the acknowledged masters of the art. Some sources even say that, while in Chaldea, he was a pupil of the great mystic, Zoroaster (Zarathustra), from whom he received the greater part of his wisdom.

In 530 BCE, he emigrated from Samos to the Italian mainland, and the colony of Magna Graecia, where he established the first of the Pythagorean enclaves at Kroton; eventually, the influence of the Brotherhood that formed around this charismatic teacher allowed them to gain supremacy over the greater part of the colony. It is said that, in certain remote valleys in southern Italy, a form of ancient Greek is still spoken, a lingering remnant of their former inhabitants. However, the dominance of the Pythagorean movement was short-lived; Pythagoras was banned from Kroton prior to his death, and the Brotherhood came to an untimely end. His disciples were sent into exile or slain, and any vestige of their presence was obliterated. Consistent with the ephemeral nature of his cult, Pythagoras left behind no personal documentation of his life and studies. The only evidence of his existence and the significance of his philosophy is provided through accounts penned by his disciples.

Although his temporal impact was brief, even prior to his death the legends about Pythagoras gradually recast him as a semi-divine being, a son of Hyperborean Apollo himself. What did survive his passing, however, was the singular vision of the universe that he propagated in his teachings:

> the Pythagorean vision of the world was so enduring, that it still permeates our thinking, even our vocabulary. The very term "philosophy" is Pythagorean in origin; so is the word "harmony" in its broader sense… in its all-embracing, unifying character; it unites religion and science, mathematics and music, medicine and cosmology, body, mind and spirit in an inspired and luminous synthesis… But the simplest approach (to it) is through music.[5]

Pythagorean Number Theory and Music

One of the earliest explications of the extraordinary Pythagorean conception of the nature of physical reality being organized according to principles of number, and the relationship of those numerological architectonics both to musical tone and the structure of the cosmos, was provided by the later Greek philosopher, Aristotle, in his *Metaphysics*:

> Since of these [mathematical] principles numbers are by nature the first, and in numbers they [the Pythagoreans] seemed to see many resemblances to the things that exist and come into being…they say that the attributes and ratios of the musical scales were expressible in numbers; since, then, all other things seemed in their whole nature to be modeled after numbers, and numbers seemed to be the first things in the whole of nature, they supposed the elements of numbers to be the elements of all things, and the whole heaven to be a musical scale and number.[6]

It is difficult for us to envision such a singular paradigm, one which presupposes a universal harmony of proportion that informs not only the infinite manifestations of physical form which surround us in our daily existence, but also aspects of that same existence which are purely immanent, chief among which were the perceptible, but intangible, vibrations of music:

> It is clear that the Pythagoreans did not simply discern congruities among number and music and the cosmos; they identified them. Music *was* number, and the cosmos *was* music. Consequently, the precepts of music as they were eventually formulated by Pythagoras were of

paramount importance, for they governed the whole scope of the perceptible and even the imperceptible universe.[7]

The crucial component of the Pythagorean corpus of theories relating to music was that, given the above, it was not to be employed, or enjoyed, merely for esthetic reasons; rather, the Master regarded music as having an authentically spiritual dimension, and he trained his followers to employ music as a healing art, for purposes of personal transformation, and to similarly treat the disharmonies that manifested in the physical body as disease.

Healing with Sound

> The healing power Pythagoras used was that of Sound itself—sound used as a power of harmonization. To harmonize in the Greek sense was to deal with the unceasing process of change that is life itself, to make this change resonant with the rhythmic flow of universal change. The universe was not seen as a static whole, but rather...a dynamic process of rhythmic formation and transformation.[8]

Pythagoras' biographer Porphyry tells us that Pythagoras "soothed the passions of the soul and body by rhythms, songs and incantations. These he adapted and applied to his friends." One of the most famous anecdotes concerning the Master is related by Iamblichus, a student of Porphyry's; I like to think of this as describing a Pythagorean musical "intervention":

> Among the deeds of Pythagoras likewise, it is said, that once through the spondaic song of a piper, he extinguished the rage of a Tauromenian lad, who had been feasting by night, and intended to burn the vestibule of his mistress, in consequence of seeing her coming from the house of his rival. For the lad was inflamed and excited [to this rash attempt] by a Phrygian song; which however Pythagoras most rapidly suppressed. But Pythagoras, as he was astronomizing, happened to meet with the Phrygian piper at an unseasonable time of night, and persuaded him to change his Phrygian for a spondaic song; through which the fury of the lad being immediately repressed, he returned home in an orderly manner, though a little before this, he could not be in the least restrained, nor would in short, bear any admonition; and even stupidly insulted Pythagoras when he met him.[9]

The Tetraktys

Let us now, in our exploration of Pythagorean number theory, return to the tetraktys, depicted in Figure 1.4.

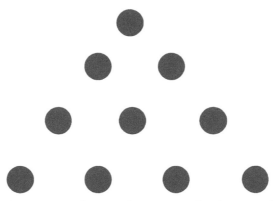

Figure 1.4 *The tetraktys was a fundamental construct of Pythagorean number theory*

The Tetraktys [also known as the decad] is an equilateral triangle formed from the sequence of the first ten numbers aligned in four rows. It is both a mathematical idea and a metaphysical symbol that embraces within itself—in seedlike form—the principles of the natural world, the harmony of the cosmos, the ascent to the divine, and the mysteries of the divine realm. So revered was this ancient symbol that it inspired ancient philosophers to swear by the name of the one who brought this gift to humanity—Pythagoras.

Attributed to Iamblichus[10]

The Significance of the Tetraktys

- The tetraktys symbolized the four elements: earth, air, fire, and water.

- These first four numbers also illustrated the harmony of the spheres and the cosmos.

- The first four numbers added up to ten, which was unity of a higher order, the first octave of the primordial creative matrix, represented by the number one.

◈   Finally, the tetraktys represented a paradigm for the emergence of consensus reality out of nothingness.

- •   The first row represented zero dimensions (a point); we can regard this as relating to the primal cosmic union, however you wish to name it, in that timeless moment of serene, perpetual stasis that was brought to an abrupt cessation by the Big Bang or its metaphysical equivalent—the Ain Soph, the Wu Ji, the Pythagorean monad, the Logos, etc. Every creation myth stipulates that the universe had its origin as a unitary generative matrix, usually female, complete and whole in and of itself, perfect, and timeless. These are essential attributes of divinity.

- •   The second row represented one dimension (a line, consisting of two points); at some critical juncture, this primordial entity embarks upon a process of self-discovery and precipitates a schism within itself, sundering its original being into two discrete polar opposites—Yin/Yang, dark/light, feminine/ masculine, *et al*. Thus, considerations of balance, proportion, harmony, relationship, etc., become paramount, and the way is prepared for the emergence of the realm of matter.

- •   The third row represented two dimensions (a plane, defined by a regular polygon of three points, a triangle); in the natural world, when the two polarities meet and unite, something new and unprecedented comes about. Usually this is the birth of new life, and here we witness the creative impetus at work. It is arguable that all great art arises from the blending of disparate elements.

    What invariably comes to mind is the concept of *chiaroscuro*, the intermingling of light (chiaro) and dark (scuro), which was a hallmark of painting in the Italian Renaissance. A similar philosophy underscores the vocal art of Italian *bel canto*, beautiful singing, which had its origins in the Baroque period. A beautiful voice must embrace and effortlessly commingle its twin registers, chest and head, throughout the entire compass of its range. It is this synergy that makes it possible for singers to essay the vocal demands of the masterpieces of the Western vocal tradition, particularly opera.

- The fourth row represented three dimensions (a triangular pyramid defined by four points); four is the number of the recognizable structures of material reality. If, for example, we look at our homes—they are bounded upon all sides by four walls, in which, at regular intervals, appear apertures which are four-sided (windows); the building itself contains subdivisions, rooms, which are usually rectangular. Upon many of the walls of these rooms are artistic renderings, usually rectangular. The computer upon which I am typing at the moment has a four-sided screen; it represents an advance upon the earlier communications technology of the book, which is similarly rectangular shaped. We house these books upon rectangular-shaped bookshelves or in a rectangular-shaped cabinet. We consume our regular meals at tables that are four-sided; we watch television on a rectangular screen, etc. Myriad other examples could be cited. Consequently, four-ness is the energy of manifestation, and we generally organize our physical space in four-square allotments. We can witness the process of transformation of a two-dimensional triangle into a three-dimensional construct, a pyramid, by the addition of the fourth point and a third, vertical, axis.

The Pythagorean musical system was likewise based on the tetraktys, as the rows can be read in successive ordered pairs (from bottom to top) as the ratios of 4:3, 3:2, 2:1, forming the basic intervals of the Pythagorean scales, which were later adopted by Western musical theorists. Pythagorean scales are based on pure, perfect fifths (produced by vibratory resonators whose dimensions are in a 3:2 proportion) and fourths (in a 4:3 ratio). These two stable, optimally blending intervals—inversions of each other, i.e., the two intervals subsume, between them, the entire frequency range of an octave—are considered harmonious and labeled "consonances" in the parlance of music theory.

Similarly, the ratios of 1:1 and 2:1 generate even more stable and harmonious intervals, i.e., the unison and the octave; these are the musical intervals with which we will be working in Vibrational Acupuncture™ treatment protocols. These latter intervals are of a higher order of consonance than the perfect fifth and fourth because they encode vibrations which, although they are, in fact, of different Hz—i.e., each subsequent octave tone is twice the frequency of the preceding, lower, octave—can be identified by the human ear as possessing an identical quality of "pitch class," i.e., A, C# (C sharp), Eb (E flat), etc. This is a concept which is known as *octave equivalence*, and the effect is to permit the processing of a myriad of different frequencies using the same set of auditory receptors within the ear and brain. In other words, we utilize the same auditory mechanisms to identify each member of an octave set, i.e., all C#s, in effect, sound the same to us, or, at the least, they are classified as being identical for purposes of identification and processing.

Music Is Number

It should be stated that the ratios that inform these musical relationships are readily manifest in the natural world; however, it was Pythagoras who, according to legend, discovered the arithmetical relationships of the two tones involved in the harmonic intervals that he and his followers had already identified as significant in their understanding of musical theory. Here is Iamblichus' version of the story:

> Intently considering once, and reasoning with himself, whether it would be possible to devise a certain instrumental assistance to the hearing, which should be firm and unerring—thus considering, as he was walking near a brazier's shop, he heard from a certain divine casualty the hammers [eating out a piece of iron on an anvil, and producing sounds that accorded with each other, one combination only excepted. But he recognized, in those sounds, the diapason, the diapente, and the diatessaron,[11] harmony... Being delighted, therefore, to find that the thing which he was anxious to discover had succeeded to his wishes by divine assistance, he went into the brazier's shop, and found by various experiments, that the difference of sound arose from the magnitude of the hammers...[12]

The essential truth revealed in this tale of Pythagoras' encounter with the blacksmiths and their inadvertently harmonious music of hammer and anvil is that there is a precise correspondence between the esthetic, and seemingly arbitrary, symphony of musical tone and the abstract, yet concrete, totality of numbers.

The musical intervals produced by the hammers were exactly equivalent to the ratios between the hammers' weights. In other words, the six-pound hammer and the twelve-pound hammer, having a weight ratio of 1:2, produced a perfect octave. The eight-pound hammer and the twelve-pound hammer, having a ratio of 2:3, produced a major fifth interval; and the nine-pound hammer and the twelve-pounder (with a 3:4 ratio), when struck simultaneously, produced a perfect fourth.

Kitty Ferguson suggests that this undoubtedly apocryphal tale may refer to the ancient mystique associated with blacksmiths.[13] They were regarded as the lineal descendants of Hephaestus (Vulcan), the smith god and primordial engineer of the Olympian pantheon. In addition to the practical skills that they offered to their communities, for example shoeing of horses, the manufacture of steel of implements as diverse as plows for tilling the soil, weapons, cookware, etc., they were also the custodians of secrets of advanced technologies, including those relating to alchemy and metallurgy, and the mathematical skills that would be required with engineering. It is generally conceded that Pythagoras was introduced to certain mystery schools during his sojourns in Egypt and India, and, following his initiation into the orders, had become privy to this arcane knowledge.

Emanations from the Ohm Tone

As we have noted above, numerical archetypes can be viewed through the model of the tetraktys as having their ultimate origin in the number one. The musical intervals that characterize most of the planetary intervals associated with the Acutonics® system, produced by specific ratios between these fundamental numbers, are likewise emanations from the fundamental of the Acutonics® planetary "scale," Ohm. Ohm resonates at a pitch of 136.1 Hz, which is approximately a C# in Western musical notation. This is illustrated in Figure 1.5.

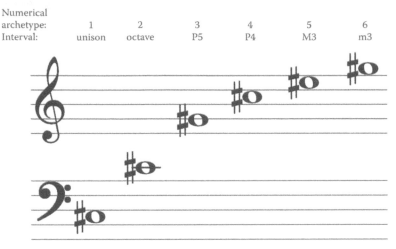

Figure 1.5 *Overtones can be regarded as emanations from the fundamental tone*

We could construe this as representing a manifestation of the intervallic "matrix" both longitudinally and temporally, in that these overtones arise in an orderly progression that only comes into being as the fundamental tone continues to resonate, although the time frame for this phenomenon is comparatively short. Another way we might view this, by confining the intervals to the octave that encompasses the Acutonics Ohm® scale, is illustrated in Figure 1.6.

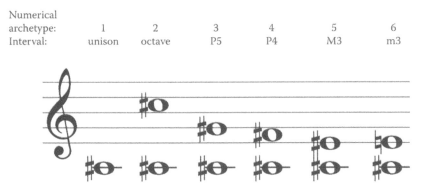

Figure 1.6 *Musical intervals arising from the Ohm overtone series*

The vertical coincidence of the intervallic tones in this model approximates the parameters within which the Acutonics® practitioner (and patient) has direct physical experience of these intervals, as a combination of two tuning forks (although we see only one pitch notated in the unison, it is produced by two identical resonators, Ohm forks). The practitioner is reminded that we will only be concerning ourselves with the first two of these intervals and tuning fork combinations; the two intervals are the most harmonious that can occur in music, the unison and octave.

Each of the intervals arising from a fundamental tone can be readily viewed as a departure from a preexisting ground state, signified by the Ohm tone; as such, they encode energetic potentials. We could categorize the paired notes of the interval as twin magnetic poles; with greater vibratory proximity, associated with a corresponding diminishment of the frequency range between the two notes, the apparent strength of the effect increases and the more highly charged, i.e., the more *dissonant*, the interval itself. The greater vibratory intensity that is characteristic of less harmonious intervals has definite applications in a therapeutic setting, but we will not capitalize upon this in the treatment protocols of Vibrational Acupuncture™. The electrical charge of acupuncture needles will engender similar effects.

The Structures of Music Are an Expression of Natural Laws

This may have seemed an extraordinarily long digression into concepts that are, to most of you, abstract at best. What possible use can this information be to you, the practitioner, who may or may not be a musician? This is to return to the argument advanced at the outset of this chapter; but, I assure you that you do not need to master this material to be effective in your application of the treatment protocols you will learn from us in this book.

Nevertheless, both of us have been resolute in our conviction, since we first began teaching our *Facial Soundscapes*™ vibrational tuning fork facial seminars, that practitioners of sound healing protocols should at least be introduced to these theoretical concepts, if only to provide reasoned arguments for your advocacy of this modality when confronting patients who are invested both in the prevailing philosophical paradigms of early-21st-century Earth and its all-pervasive lower vibration music:

> Its effect upon the soul is to make nigh-impossible the true inner silence and peace necessary for the contemplation of eternal verities. How

necessary it is in this age for *some* to have the courage to…separate themselves from the pack who long ago sold their lives and personalities to this sound.[14]

What is immediately apparent from an exploration of Pythagorean number theory and its eventual incorporation into the musical theory of the West is that, like the Chinese, the ancient Greeks were well acquainted with the potential power of music to exercise an influence for good or ill. The members of the Pythagorean Brotherhood, following the shining example of their founder, prioritized the playing of music as being for healing purposes. However, the secrets of this unitary vision of a harmonious cosmos, and the transformative application of the planetary frequencies divined by the Master, were not to be imparted willy-nilly to all and sundry; they were only revealed to aspirants following their movement through a rigidly demarcated three-tiered system of apprenticeship and education. Only after the acolyte had become sufficiently evolved through repeated exposure to the ideal proportions of the musical intervals, and other practices designed to heighten their consciousness, would they then be qualified to extend the benefits of this knowledge to others.

> Through foolishness they deceived themselves into thinking that there was no right or wrong in music—that it was to be judged good or bad by the pleasure it gave. By their work and their theories, they infected the masses with the presumption to think themselves adequate judges… As it was the criterion was not music, but a reputation for promiscuous cleverness and a spirit of law-breaking.

Plato, in the above quote from his dialogue *Laws*, could have been describing the worldwide hegemony of popular music that has consolidated its presence for the past 50 years, with its emphasis on "sex, drugs, and rock and roll," and the corrosive impact it has had upon culture and the social maturation of the individual. We are presently inhabiting a world in which the kind of tonal anarchy that these philosopher musicians, from East and West, would have dreaded, is omnipresent.

Moreover, the worldwide culture is dominated in its thinking by the great secular religion, science, which, ironically, emerged for the first time concurrent with the rediscovery of much of the esoteric knowledge of the Hellenic world by Europeans. As modern acolytes of this ancient knowledge of numbers and proportions, and possessing the skills of energy healers, you will be able to impart the transformative vibrations embodied in the perfect harmonies of the unison and octave of the primal Acutonics® Earth tone, Ohm, to your patients, in synergy with very sophisticated acupuncture needling.

However, it is likely that you will encounter those patients who will be skeptical of the significance of the sound-healing component of this innovative modality, Vibrational Acupuncture™. These individuals may, in fact, be devotees of any number of forms of what we can only term, based upon the criteria of these estimable teachers, degenerate music. They may scoff at the notion that these cosmic tones will have any beneficial effect upon their energetic systems—thoroughly discombobulated by the disharmonious music with which they surround themselves, and the deleterious impact of their lifestyle choices. This being said, it may be that they will consent to the gentle ministrations of these harmonious tuning fork combinations and find that they are changed by their experience.

We have witnessed this in the past: we were teaching a seminar in Calgary, Alberta, Canada, and one of the participants was an M.D. who administered an enormously successful acupuncture pain clinic. As a physician, she was, naturally, a proponent of the prevailing scientific, rational world view and scornful in her contempt for what she perceived to be the "airy-fairy" nature of tuning forks. She did, however, agree to experience the Grounding Protocol with Ohm Unison to which you will be introduced later in the book. The results were dramatic: she marveled at the effect. In fact, upon merely hearing the Ohm tone, her entire demeanor changed. She became an instant convert.

There will be those, however, resolute in their scientific convictions, who will give no credence to such a modality. Therefore, if there is one concept that I urge you to take away from this chapter, it is the following, which I will reiterate from above: "The structures of music are an expression of natural laws." You can inform these individuals that the 2:1 frequency relationship of the octave is as much a universal constant as the law of gravity, or Einstein's famous dictum: $E = mc^2$. Pure Pythagorean musical intervals exist in the same sort of rarified conceptual universe as any abstruse mathematical theorem. This viewpoint is echoed by Lyndon Larouche, Jr., in his article "The science of music: Solution to Plato's paradox of the one and the many":

Such fundamentally characteristic features of natural music such as 1) *bel canto* vocalization, 2) voice-registration, and 3) a well-tempered scale with middle C set at approximately 256 cycles are biologically determined, and thus inherent truths of existence predating the first physicist.[15]

I will remind you of the comparison I offered at the outset of this chapter, the parallels between musical tone, the bedrock of harmony, and the atom, the building block of the elements that comprise our universe. The analogy is not merely one of proportional structures, electrons, and overtones, but likewise of oscillating particles and waves. Ancient peoples anticipated the discoveries of 20th-century scientific endeavor in their advocacy of a vibrational paradigm of creation. Most scientists will acknowledge the fact that the apparent unyielding and impermeable nature of solid reality is entirely illusory—that, beneath the surface of a table, for instance, the constituent atoms of the molecules that have combined to produce its structure, whether it be wood, plastic, or metal, are constantly in motion. What is this, if not a confirmation of the ultimately vibratory nature of reality?

If such a "substantial" product of human technological endeavor is merely a manifestation of vibrating submolecular particles in a particular array, how much more so the fragile architecture of the human body? In engaging with it with instruments that are intrinsic to its nature, tuned planetary resonators, we have the capacity to effect healing at the most profound of levels. The combined impact of these two ancient systems of healing, Chinese medicine with its poetic and energetic landscape of points and meridians, and Pythagorean-style planetary sound therapy, is tremendous in its synergy.

The watery vibrations of healing sound can traverse the totality of the structure of our bodies to effect beneficial change at the primal level of organization, DNA. One of the principal means we will utilize to address this vital aspect of our being is through treating the points of the Eight Extraordinary meridians of Chinese medicine, to which you will be introduced in Chapter 3.

The Cosmos Is Music: The Music of the Spheres (in Brief)

> The key, in this tradition, to the ordering of the cosmos, whether astronomically or musically, is of course number – a discovery which was transmitted to Western thinkers by Pythagoras. Indeed...number determines all things in nature and their concrete manifestation, together with all rhythms and cycles of life.[16]

The philosophers of the pre-modern world perceived the universe as being essentially harmonious in nature. These leading lights of Eastern and Western thought acknowledged that, in an ideal world, human existence should mirror the orderly arrangement of the heavens by whatever means possible and sought to recreate these conditions in the arrangement of their cities, the structures of their temples, etc. A notable architectural example of this is the Great Pyramid complex of the Giza Plateau in Upper Egypt, which has been demonstrated by paleo-archeologists to align significantly with stars in the belt of the constellation Orion, the Hunter, although this theory is disputed by orthodox Egyptologists. A similar orientation can be discerned in the philosophy of Chinese medicine, in which the perennial cycle of the seasons here on Earth finds its echo in the elemental structure not only of nature, but also of human beings. Western medicine, originally based in astrology, likewise regarded the human body as being a microcosm, a reflection, in incarnate form, of the heavens.

In the West, Pythagoras was the first proponent of a model of celestial harmony, the Music of the Spheres, in which planetary motion was responsible for the production of actual musical tones. He postulated that the seven planets of the Greek solar system—Sun, Moon, Mercury, Venus, Mars, Jupiter, and Saturn—as they orbited Earth, in a geocentric array, did so in perfect crystalline spheres, and this regular movement elicited the heavenly sounds: "In the Platonic/Pythagorean tradition, music and the stars are inextricably linked as audible and visible images of an invisible dimension of existence, whose intellectual perception is made possible through the senses of hearing and sight."[17]

While his disciples fervently believed that Pythagoras, because of his semi-divine nature, could actually perceive these supernal harmonies, a key element of his approach to sound healing was the recreation of the planetary music here on Earth. To this end, he reconfigured the Greek lyre, which had seven strings, to become a delivery system for the appropriate frequencies; its tones, tuned to a cosmic scale of his own devising, were considered to replicate the sound of the planets traversing their crystalline spheres. This Pythagorean practice of healing with planetary sound might arguably be said to be a kind of proto-music therapy, in which soothing musical sounds, apprehended by the ear, can effect beneficial changes in the human "instrument."

In the intervening centuries following his death and the purging of his followers, Pythagoras' idea of celestial harmony received many notable reinterpretations, in particular by Plato, who devotes an entire section of his book, *Timaeus*, to the creation of the universe along Pythagorean musical lines by means of the overtone series. However, subsequent to the collapse of the Roman Empire in the late 5th century and the descent of the long night of comparative intellectual ignorance and Christian religious superstition labeled the Dark Ages, knowledge of these teachings went into eclipse for many centuries.

It was only with the partial re-emergence of the intellectual legacy of the Hellenic world that occurred in the later Middle Ages, precipitated in the 12th century by the Medieval Scholastics with their advocacy of Aristotelian philosophy, that the eventual rediscovery of the Platonic oeuvre became possible. In the Renaissance, his major works were translated into Latin by the polymath Marsilio Ficino—Christian priest, astrologer, herbalist, magician, and musician—at the behest of Cosimo de' Medici, who had decided to reinstitute the Platonic Academy in his own city of Florence. Ficino later propagated his own version of healing with astrological music in his writings.

The contemporary awareness of Plato's interpretation of Pythagoras' singular vision of cosmic harmony that arose in the wake of Ficino's efforts served, in the subsequent centuries, to inspire many great minds. Among them was the brilliant 17th-century German astronomer Johannes Kepler, who, like many of his peers, including Galileo and Copernicus, saw no inherent conflict between the integrative world view of ancient philosophy and the emergent scientific paradigm. Motivated by these venerable teachings, Kepler the metaphysician formulated his own theories of heavenly music in his treatise *Die Harmonie der Welt*.

More pertinent to our discussion is the fact that Kepler, in his role as scientist, benefiting from exacting observations of planetary positions performed and catalogued by a team of his colleagues working under the patronage of the wealthy Danish astronomer Tycho Brahe, was, for the first time, able to arrive at a theoretical construct for the configuration of planetary orbits in a heliocentric solar system. In 1609, he published the results of his findings in the first two laws of planetary motion, adding a third nearly a decade later in 1618. It was the first of his laws that obviated the previous model of circular orbits, originally formulated by the Hellenic astronomer/astrologer Claudius Ptolemy, in the 2nd century CE.

Ironically, although a devotee of the Pythagorean world view, through his discoveries he drove the final metaphorical nail into the Greek philosopher's coffin, laying to rest his theoretical mechanism for the generation of celestial harmony. He affirmed the scientific rectitude of the heliocentric model of his contemporary Copernicus, and posited that the planets revolve around the Sun, not in Pythagoras' crystalline spheres, but rather in elliptical orbits: "There may exist other harmonic laws, unnoticed by astronomers, which may concern the speeds of the planets' movements in their orbits. Literally, these speeds on the harmonic level, would represent the planets' pitch frequencies."[18]

Some 300-plus years later, in 1978, the Pythagorean vision of heavenly music and personal transformation was notably resuscitated in the innovative application of modern astronomical knowledge to this age-old paradigm, by Swiss mathematician and musicologist Hans Cousto. In his groundbreaking book, *The Cosmic Octave*, capitalizing upon contemporary understanding of planetary orbits made possible by the discoveries of Kepler and others, he offers a simple, but radical, mathematical formula for the conversion of the motion of the planets of the expanded solar system, including Uranus, Neptune, and Pluto, plus Earth (and other planetary and cosmic cycles), into musical frequency. This derivation of tone from planetary movement is a fulfillment of, and a profound expansion upon, the original Pythagorean paradigm, and it engenders an entirely new spectrum of planetary sounds.

> it was the result of a way of seeing things that moved me to combine the old teachings of harmonics with new finds in physics and other sciences...with which it is possible to transpose the movements of the planets into audible rhythms and sounds.[19]

In order to bring these newly calculated cosmic frequencies to bear upon the human instrument, in alignment with the traditions of Pythagorean music therapy, Cousto devised and manufactured his own instruments to make them accessible to human hearing, an assemblage of planetary tuning forks. These healing tools can be said to "embody" Pythagoras' celestial harmonies and function as archetypal distillations of the essence of the planets themselves. The derivation of precise frequencies for each planet from its orbital period in seconds grounds the theoretical edifice of Pythagoras' musical spheres firmly in contemporary scientific and mathematical reality.

Although a theoretician, and not a healer, Cousto further anchors the therapeutic use of cosmic music here on Earth; *The Cosmic Octave* delineates rudimentary guidelines for how his planetary tuning forks may be employed upon the body via acupuncture points. In so doing, he was instrumental in revitalizing the Pythagorean vibratory healing philosophy for late-20th-century healthcare practitioners, providing an avenue to an authentically somatic system of planetary healing.

It remained then for Donna Carey, L.Ac., visionary co-creator of the Acutonics® sound healing system and an acupuncturist versed in the Western esoteric traditions, to further integrate planetary tuning forks modeled after Cousto's, tuned to his planetary frequencies, within a constitutional body treatment protocol, utilizing the points and meridians of Chinese medicine. In her adoption of the planetary tonal framework outlined in *The Cosmic Octave* for the Acutonics® healing system, Carey designated the principal one of Cousto's three Earth tones as Ohm, that which he designated as Earth-Year (his terminology is "Om"), with a calculated frequency of 136.1 Hz. It became the central frequency of the Acutonics® vibrational healing paradigm.

Earth Is Indeed at the Center ——————————————

Those enterprising pioneers of the fledging astronomical science in the Renaissance—Kepler, Galileo, Brahe, Copernicus, and others— were, through their discoveries, responsible for dislodging our planet from its privileged position at the center of the universe, demoting it to a diminished existence as just another planetary body, by no means the largest, orbiting a small yellow star at the outer fringes of an enormous galaxy.

However, despite our intellectual awareness of this altered heliocentric reality, verified by our species' explorations of the solar system in recent decades, when we gaze out from our orbiting observational observatory, *terra firma*, at the heavens, as did our primordial ancestors, we witness the same cosmos. We are surrounded on all sides by those titanic stellar groupings, the constellations, vastly remote, yet vibrant in their archetypal resonance, the embodiment of collective experience expressed through myths from around the world. Simultaneously, traversing the limitless depths of starry space, those seven perennial wanderers, the planets, known to the West and elsewhere, continue faithfully in their circumnavigation of the sky, marking the ongoing increments of cosmic time.

To our all-too-human eyes, Earth remains at the center...just as it was in the traditional schema of the Five Elements, according to the Chinese, denizens of Middle Earth, and in the astrological art of the West, the other theoretical linchpin of Vibrational Acupuncture™. This venerable planetary science remains steadfastly geocentric in its orientation, for it is here on Earth that we dwell and live out the finite span of our mortal existence. Thus, it is appropriate that the Acutonics® sound healing system, too, which is informed by Western astrological archetypes, is similarly Earth-centered from a *tonal* perspective.

> *The entire world is a musical instrument, the pole of the world celestial is intersected where this heavenly chord is divided by the spiritual sun. Earthly music is an echo of this cosmic harmony; it is a relic of heaven.*
>
> Author unknown

Additionally, extrapolating from the information provided by Cousto in *The Cosmic Octave*, it can be attested that the gamut of planetary frequencies that may be calculated by means of his energy equation may be regarded as overtones of his fundamental Earth tone, 136.1 Hz. This further underscores the relevance of an Earth-centered harmony to this revitalized approach to Pythagorean-style planetary sound healing.

With all this in mind, let us now consider the various archetypal underpinnings of the Acutonics Ohm® Earth-Year tone.

The Myth of Earth

From my perspective as a Western astrologer, the influence of the Greco-Roman paradigm of the cosmos remains paramount in our consideration of planetary archetypes. One cannot overestimate the continuing impact of a particular nomenclature upon the psyche and temperament of a people. From an esoteric perspective, names embody vital characteristics, both numerologically and linguistically, and they may have a demonstrable impact upon a person's destiny; a derogatory or otherwise unfortunate name can become a source of ridicule or censure, even persecution. The decision to elect a name of personal significance for oneself, to slough off one that is considered less than desirable, is often a gesture of profound empowerment, helping the person to overcome previous impediments.

In the same manner, the names of the planets and other features of the heavens, a vital aspect of the linguistic heritage of those great Mediterranean civilizations, retain their relevance in contemporary languages; in English, for example, we still describe individuals as having personalities that are mercurial, martial, jovial, saturnine, etc. This nomenclature likewise extends to other Romance languages. People who are aberrant mentally are lunatics, subject to the irrational effects of the Moon, Luna. Those persons who have accumulated a great deal of money, and who use it to advance their aims, remain plutocrats, because Pluto, the god of the underworld, over time became associated with the riches, i.e., gold and silver, that are housed deep within the bosom of the Earth. There is a myriad of other examples that I could present for your consideration.

Hence, while, as we shall see below, human beings have worshipped a plenitude of earth goddesses, found in every corner of the globe, and fashioned an associated wealth of myths associated with these powerful female deities, we will confine ourselves for the purposes of this volume to one myth, a colorful Greek story that pertains to the original denizens of Earth and sky, Gaea and Uranus.

Gaea, The Divine Mother

> In the older mother myths and rites, the light and darker aspects of the mixed thing that is life had been honored equally and together… Where the goddess had been venerated as the giver and supporter of life as well as consumer of the dead, women as her representatives had been accorded a paramount position in society as well as in cult.[20]

Gaea was the great creative progenitrix of the early Greeks. She was considered the embodiment of Earth itself and worshipped for her abundant fecundity, by means of which she engendered the whole of nature and the gods and goddesses of the Greek pantheon, through her birthing of the first "humanoid" beings, the Titans.

In Hesiod's *Theogony*, the creation story of the ancient Greeks, composed sometime in the 7th century BCE, the only extant being in the universe is Chaos, composed of equal parts of void, mass, and darkness, intermingled in roiling confusion—a primordial cosmological stew. Consistent with the majority of creation myths around the world, the initial creative activity in the *Theogony* is that of parthenogenesis; miraculously, out of chaos, Gaea comes into existence, and, in short order, while in a dormant state, i.e., "in her sleep," this undifferentiated feminine matrix undergoes a type of mitosis, reproduction without *eros*,[21] splitting off from herself the starry heavens, Uranus, and the sea, Pontus. In this manner, creation arranges itself according to the customary three-tiered paradigm, later echoed in the Greek pantheon as Zeus (sky), Poseidon (sea), and Hades (underworld); the disappearance of a feminine energy from this Olympian triumvirate is consistent with later mythic developments.

> The ancient Great Mother of All Living gave birth parthenogenetically to herself and the entire cosmos. She was the world egg, containing the two halves of all polarities or dualisms – the Yin/Yang of continuity and change, expansion and contraction of the universe. This process is symbolized by the spiral turning continuously in and on itself, by conscious breath waking from sleep and sinking back into sleep.[22]

In due course, Uranus, by default the god of the sky, becomes Gaea's consort. This elemental couple are thereafter conjoined in an intimate bond that rendered the earth goddess endlessly fertile, perpetually showered by the sky god with life-giving floods of rain. As ancient peoples observed, the vaulted realm of the sky surrounded the globe of Earth on all sides, wrapping her in a tender embrace. In her connubial bliss, inseminated by her male counterpart, Gaea effortlessly populated the entire terrestrial sphere with every imaginable type of creature, in an abundant and endlessly variegated cavalcade of life.

Some sources, such as authors Marija Gimbutas and Barbara Walker,[23] maintain that Gaea as Mother Earth is a Greek avatar of a pre-Indo-

European Great Mother who had been venerated in Neolithic times, in a widespread matrifocal culture. However, despite the precedent for their speculations in the writings of Joseph Campbell, these theories remain controversial in orthodox archaeological circles.

The idea that the fertile earth itself is female, nurturing mankind, and the anthropomorphic conversion of our planet into a mother goddess, was not limited to the Mediterranean. The influence of Sumerian mythology can clearly be discerned in the account of darkness on the face of the Deep, referring to oceanic depths, in the first chapter of Genesis; this parallels the identification of the earlier Babylonian goddess Tiamat with the watery Abyss, the primordial sea.

The title "the mother of life" was later given to the Akkadian goddess Kubau, and hence to Hurrian Hepa, emerging as Hebrew Eve (Heva) and Phrygian Kubala (Cybele). In Norse mythology, the Great Mother, the mother of the thunder god, Thor himself, was known as Jord, Hlódyn, or Fjörgyn. The Irish Celts worshipped Danu, whereas the Welsh Celts worshipped Dôn; the predominance of place names throughout Europe that would appear derivative of these linguistic antecedents, such the Danube River, Don River, Dnieper River, Danzig, etc., are strongly suggestive of a common origin, lending credence to the idea of a ubiquitous, proto-Indo-European mother goddess. In Lithuanian mythology, Gaea-Žemė is the daughter of the Sun and the Moon; she is also the consort of Dangus (also known as Varuna; this epithet is demonstrably a cognate of Uranus, and Varuna is likewise the Vedic sky god).

In Pacific cultures, the Earth Mother assumed as many guises and a similar plethora of archetypal attributes among the diverse cultures who revered her; for example, the creation myth of the Māori features the Earth Mother, Papatūānuku, partner to Ranginui, the Sky Father. In the Andes mountain ranges of South America, a belief concerning the Pachamama still persists in certain regions of Bolivia, Peru, Ecuador, Argentina, and Chile. The origin of the name is the Quechua word "Pacha," meaning "change" or "epoch," linked with "Mama," meaning "mother." Ancient Mexican cultures referred to mother Earth as Tonantzin Tlalli, meaning "Revered Mother Earth." In the Hindu religion, the mother of all creation is called Gayatri; there is undoubtedly a linguistic and cultural linkage between she and Gaea, mirroring the demonstrable connection of Uranus and Varuna.

Unlike her "grandson," Olympian Zeus, a roving nomad god of the open sky, like her consort Uranus, Gaea was manifest in enclosed spaces: the house, the courtyard, the womb, the cave. Her sacred animals are the serpent, the lunar bull, the pig, and bees.

Archetypal Qualities of Earth

- Maternal instincts
- Origin, source
- Constancy, permanence
- Nature, the natural world
- Creativity
- Primogeniture
- Fecundity
- Abundance, ripeness
- Nurturance
- Groundedness; anchor
- Tranquility

Planetary Glyph: The Cross: Guaternity (Matter)

The cross that comprises the glyph for Earth is composed of two lines of equal length, which divide a plane into four regions. In numerology, four is the number of manifestation; three, as the union of one and two, the primal polarities, remains the determinant of a two-dimensional surface. However, when we modulate energetically from three to four, we enter the realm of materiality; a pyramid composed of four equidistant points in space becomes, in our perception, a three-dimensional solid. In contrast, an equilateral triangle, despite its perfection of proportion as a regular polygon, remains fixed in two dimensions only. A pyramid has length, breadth, and height; subsumes physical space; and possesses demonstrable mass. Our conception of the material world is thereby four-square; four is a number of wholeness and completion, an archetypal association that we find exemplified in such cultural phenomena as the four winds, seasons, elements, directions, weeks of the month, suits of the Tarot, Horsemen of the Apocalypse, and corners of the Earth.

The dwellings that most of us inhabit, either by choice or due to societal convention or constraint, as we noted above, are the equivalent of little boxes, extensions of four-square polygons into three-dimensional space. They take the form of cubes if all their dimensions are equal, or regular parallelepipeds or cuboids. We are isolated from the natural world by these fourfold material structures, and the visible artifacts of our lives, our possessions, can be likewise confined to similar box-like containers.

Carl Jung, while recuperating from a near-death experience in 1944, during which he had an extraordinary unitary vision of the round globe of Earth from thousands of miles out in space, associated his impending resumption of normal life with a return to the "box system":

> In reality, a good three weeks were still to pass before I could truly make up my mind to live again… The view of city and mountains from my sickbed seemed to me like a painted curtain with black holes in it, or a tattered sheet of newspaper full of photographs that meant nothing. Disappointed, I thought: "Now I must return to 'the box system' again."
>
> For it seemed to me as if behind the horizon of the cosmos a three-dimensional world had been artificially built up, in which each person sat by himself in a little box. And now I should have to convince myself all over again that this was important! Life and the whole world struck me as a prison, and it bothered me beyond measure that I should again be finding all that quite in order.[24]

In the early 21st century, the majority of us readily interact by electronic means with a worldwide community, utilizing devices—smartphones, tablets, televisions, laptop computers—that, through the wondrous magic of their rectangular portals, permit us contact with other lives. These miraculous technological "boxes" afford us, however, only a semblance of authentic human interaction. In a similar fashion, we gaze through the rectangular windows of our homes—and, when we temporarily escape the confines of these domiciles, through the viewing ports of our vehicles—at the splendors of nature, but we are similarly deprived of any vital experience of it. It is this energy of four that likewise constrains us on a psychospiritual level, miring us in a constant struggle for survival, rendering us relentlessly earthbound, and preventing our access to more transcendent realms of being.

As representative of physical matter, the cross illustrates our physical imperfection and frailty and the limits of our capacity to sustain ourselves in any given incarnation. All organic life-forms on this planet are subject to the dictates of a limited life span, and consciousness of our eventual mortality is the great psychic burden placed upon our species in particular. We can also view the four arms plus the center of the cross as equaling five in total, which is the number of humanity; human beings have five limbs, as one can observe most memorably in Leonardo da Vinci's portrait of Vitruvian Man, as well as in the fact that we each possess five digits on our hands and feet. In this sense, the cross also points to our potential to transcend the material plane, to evolve from the energy of four, matter, to that of five, spirit.

We can see the intersection of the two lines as coordinates, which pinpoint our existence at a specific locus in space and time. The figure also presents us with two seemingly irreconcilable polar opposites that can be seen to delineate the manifold divisions between the inhabitants of this sphere. The cross is a crossroads, a place of meeting, communication, and exchange of ideas. We can view the horizontal axis of the cross as two arms that have the potential to embrace or thrust away, once again, as illustrative of the potential for relationship or conflict.

The endpoints of the lines plot out equidistant points on the arc of a great circle, thus depicting Earth at the center of the figure, in its perennial orbit around the Sun, locating humanity within the vastness of galactic space. Finally, the lines of the cross converge and flow toward the center, the source of gravitational attraction, which anchors us here on Earth, in the realm of matter. We are subject to the pull of gravity for the entirety of our existence and only escape its inexorable tug when we leave the body to continue our soul's journey.

Musical Intervals: The Unison and the Octave ————
Consonance vs. Dissonance

The etymology of the English words "consonance" and "dissonance" originates with the Latin verb *sonare*, "to sound," prefixed by either of the contrasting prepositions *con* ("with/to") and *de* ("from"). Therefore, consonant intervals are generated by tones that sound "toward" each other; dissonant intervals sound "away from" each other, i.e., they require some kind of resolution, movement, to a consonance. It is this perceived harmonic tension that we recognize as indicating dissonance. In general, greater vibrational proximity translates into a higher level of dissonance, which can be detected as audible pulsations in the sound, known as beats; oscilloscope tracings reveal that the wave forms associated with these dissonant intervals manifest peaks of amplitude that essentially overlap. These electronically generated images provide visual evidence for the auditory perception provided by these dissonant frequency combinations. Furthermore, they validate our discomfort with such harmonies, which might otherwise be regarded as inconsequential in a culture such as ours, in which the faculty of hearing and the negative impact of discordant music are of decidedly secondary importance.

As we have stipulated above in our discussion of Quantum Music Theory, qualities of dissonance and consonance are not merely subjective,[25] and these attributes ultimately derive from the interrelationships that occur in the natural overtone series, the sequence of subsidiary tones that comprise the tonal spectrum of any musical note.

The further away from this "fundamental" tone in the overtone series, the more dissonant the interval created. For example, the tonic note of the Acutonics® system is the Earth tone Ohm, 136.1 Hz, which is approximately a C# in standard Western tuning. The first overtone of the series arising from Ohm is the C# an octave higher; the next overtone is the perfect fifth above that, G#; the next the perfect fourth above that, a C# two octaves higher than the Ohm tone, etc. Each of the intervals constructed using these succeeding overtones, i.e., the octave, the perfect fifth, and the perfect fourth, is more dissonant than the preceding one, although still perceived by our ears as consonant and defined as such.

While there are several intervals in what I refer to as the Ohm "constellation" in the Acutonics® planetary system, we are only concerned in this book with the unison and the octave.

Unison: the Ohm tone itself, 136.1 Hz, is derived from Earth's orbital period around the Sun, which takes a year, 365.25 days; Hans Cousto referred to this tone as Earth-Year. The unison partakes of the archetypal energy of the number one, as it is generated by two identical resonators sounding simultaneously, in a 1:1 frequency ratio. It is, therefore, an interval in which we can sense the primordial unity from which the universe sprang in that instant before the Big Bang. It embodies a quality of harmony and balance that is intrinsically linked with our notions of

Earth, of groundedness and connectedness. As such, this Earth tone evokes a response of calm, with a relaxed, focused awareness. The Ohm and Low Ohm tuning forks both encode this same energy at different frequency levels.

> *Octavus sanctos omnes docet esse beatos. (The eighth, the octave, teaches all the saints that they are blessed.)*
>
> Inscription found on the capitals of the abbey church at Cluny[26]

Octave: As we learned earlier in this discussion, the characteristic proportion of the octave is 2:1, which means that of the two tones that comprise this interval, one is precisely twice the frequency of the other. The Acutonics Low Ohm® tuning fork resonates at a frequency of 68.05 Hz, half that of Ohm.

If the unison represents, in its unanimity, the perfect, unchanging, self-contained essence of divinity, then the octave can be regarded as an initial differentiation of that primordial generative matrix and foundational tone, its fission into two diametrically opposed yet complementary polarities, for example, Yang and Yin. In the musical realm, however, these disparate tones remain essentially harmonious, because of the proportional relationship of their frequency, that same 2:1 ratio, which permits us to perceive them as being of the same nature.

The resounding of successive superoctaves, i.e., octaves that are higher in frequency, may be likened in this regard to the stages in an organic process of evolution and corresponding increases in consciousness. As each superoctave rises in pitch, it inhabits an increasingly rarefied presence in our sensory awareness, not least of all because it, by definition, has fewer overtones. Eventually, the octave modulation gives rise to a tone that disappears from our hearing altogether, leaving behind the realm of matter, returning to the empyrean regions of the Music of the Spheres.

The octave is a fundamental organizing principle of vibration, whether it be audible sound or visible light, although of the latter, we can only perceive a single octave with our eyes. Moreover, the 2:1 constant of the octave relationship has an interesting relevance to the solar system itself, with each successive planet being approximately twice the distance from the Sun as the preceding one, the nature of which is expressed in Bode's Law. The seven original planets of the geocentric solar system would also be regarded as comprising an octave, and this was the nature of the cosmic scale first envisioned by Pythagoras, to which he tuned the seven strings of the Greek lyre so as to make celestial music available to his disciples.

Here on Earth, an octave is naturally engendered when men and women sing a melody in unison, particularly in hymn singing; because of their different anatomical structure (as we learned previously, men have larger larynxes, and hence, longer vocal cords), men's and women's vocal cords phonate essentially one octave apart. We can view the octave as an expression of this balanced relationship and harmony between the dual archetypes of Yin and Yang, as manifested here in the sounds of men's and women's voices.

In the Acutonics® system, the octave is produced by Ohm in conjunction with Low Ohm, which sounds an octave lower than Ohm. It is therefore appropriate for us to assert that, given that the Low Ohm frequency is an octave lower than Middle Ohm, the Low Ohm Unison is probably more grounding than the Ohm Unison.

Chapter 2

~~∞o○( )○o∞~~

Practical Discernment: Tuning Forks and/or Needles?

Let yourself be drawn to those things you truly love.

Rumi

This chapter provides practical information required for Vibrational Acupuncture™ treatments. It is very important for you, the practitioner, to know when to use acupuncture needles or tuning forks, or synergize both modalities.

What Is Vibrational Acupuncture™? ————————————

In this innovative approach, Acutonics Ohm® tuning forks are employed by themselves, or in conjunction with acupuncture needles, on both the face and body. This vibrational Qi of resonant sound enters the body via acupuncture points and the meridians. This effect is enhanced by both the sound conductivity of the skeletal structure (bones) and the body's innate watery consistency. This combination facilitates the transmission of transformational vibrations throughout the body. The pervasive nature of sound vibration permits healing energy and intention to reach the deepest levels of our being; in effect, tuning fork treatments beneficially affect the DNA structure and our Jing: "Jing, best translated as Essence, is the substance that underlies all organic life. It is the source of organic change...and the basis of reproduction and development."[1]

The Resonance of Intention

The concept of resonance is closely connected to a commonality of interest, a similarity in nature or character; it is a kinship marked by an affinity to something or someone. In a healing context, exposure of a patient to the appropriate resonance precipitates a process of energetic alignment or entrainment, during which the practitioner enters into a profound rapport with the patient. This energetic vibrational framework invokes a powerful state of compassionate engagement. Lynne McTaggart makes the following observation about intention, which seems particularly apropos given one of the two treatment modalities we are highlighting in this work: "Intention appears to be something akin to a tuning fork, causing the tuning forks of all things in the universe to resonate at the same frequency."[2]

> If you are not a licensed or registered acupuncturist (or the equivalent), you are not qualified to use needles in any of the recommended treatments in this book. Use tuning forks; they are very effective and non-invasive.

Integrating Acupuncture Needles with Tuning Forks

Acupuncture needles stimulate specific acupoints along the course of the meridians. This action restores balance and encourages Qi or energy to flow to the organs and other bodily systems. As a result of this process, the body's normal homeostatic balance is restored, and the body can self-heal.

Whereas acupuncture needling enhances blood flow and induces a positive microtrauma, a minor injury to the body that mobilizes its immune response, the vibratory Qi of tuning forks gently flows and resonates throughout the body via the bone structure, the Kidney meridian, and the Water element.

Together, the two modalities balance Yin and Yang, both calm and stimulate, and simultaneously ground and lift up the Qi. This permits the integration of Water/Fire polarities within the body, allowing for a flow of Shen spirit in physical form and contributing to the manifestation of one's particular destiny. One of the tenets of Western alchemy was that spirit was trapped in the realm of matter, and the goal of the alchemical *opus* was to liberate that spirit. Paradoxically, however, it is only through spirit's descent into matter that it may experience the manifold blessings of life in physical form, and thereby advance its own evolution on a conscious level. Therefore, in seeking to manifest a singular destiny in a given life, we, as containers for this divine essence, provide spirit with the capacity to learn more of itself.

Tuning forks impart sound waves to the body as an adaptogen; therefore, the body will only absorb the resonance it requires. The frequencies transmitted by tuning forks directly impact the Water element, and, by extension, the Kidney essence and bone marrow. In addition to their movement along the recognizable energy channels of the acupuncture meridians, healing sound vibrations can travel to every cell of the body via an embedded network of water channel proteins or *aquaporins*. These specialized structures facilitate the transfer of water molecules across the cellular membrane, permitting each individual cell to receive the necessary hydration and nutrients, and thereafter to eliminate the by-products of its metabolism.

We are accustomed to associating the faculty of hearing only with the ears, which function as collectors of ambient sound waves for interpretation by the brain. However, it can be readily demonstrated that, given a resonator of sufficient amplitude, the ensuing vibrations can be perceived and experienced with the entire body; for example, were you to stand sufficiently close to an amplifier during a rock concert, not only would your ears be overwhelmed by the sheer volume of the music, in ranges up to almost 130 decibels at times, louder than a chainsaw, but you would also feel the vibrations emitted by the amplified sound throughout your anatomy. We should note, as well, that deaf people similarly process music in the area of the brain that is associated with hearing.[3] They sense vibration with their bodies and can interact with hearing musicians based upon this alternative sensory input; a notable example of this is the extraordinary Scottish classical percussionist Dame Evelyn Glennie, who performs regularly with symphony orchestras while in bare feet, by means of which she can detect the rhythms of the music.

In a similar fashion, the access to the minutest constituents of our physical being, single cells, afforded to water molecules through the agency of the ubiquitous aquaporins means that every cell of the body functions as a little "ear." Consequently, in treating a patient, the practitioner may direct transformative planetary and other frequencies with intention to effect change at the fundamental level of organization.

Acu-Sound Treatment Guidelines

Use tuning forks if a patient presents with any of the following symptoms.

◈ Needle-phobic with sensitivity issues.

◈ Adrenally exhausted; on overload and "running on empty," like a car without gasoline.

◈ Hypervigilant, with a history of abuse or violence.

◈ Severely energy (Qi) deficient.

◈ Immune deficiency, chronic fatigue, fibromyalgia, lupus, etc.

◈ Hemophilia, i.e., patients who bleed and bruise easily if needled.

◈ Ungrounded, restless, unreceptive patients, for example, those with attention deficit disorder (ADD), hyperactive children, and people with an inability to concentrate/focus, learning disorders, and Down's syndrome.

◈ A marked preference for sound and not needles; be advised that the patient may not know why they prefer sound. Honor their wishes.

◈ Tuning forks are especially effective in the treatment of children, animals, the elderly, and sensitive souls.

Acupuncture Needles Move Qi and Are Electrical in Effect

The impact of acupuncture needling is primarily electrical; piercing the body, as noted previously, can cause a beneficial microtrauma, which energizes, moves, and unblocks Qi. Acupuncture needles act as a "lightning rod," or an antenna, that attracts universal Qi to the area punctured. Acupuncture points and meridians correspond to fascia, which conducts electricity (see "Fascia Talk" in Chapter 3).

Use acupuncture needles in the following instances.

◈ The patient believes that acupuncture needling is more effective than sound vibration.

◈ The patient is very Yang or excess, and responds better if needles are retained in the body for a longer period of time.

⟐ They have a sports-related injury and want to experience the cathartic release of the muscles involved.

⟐ Particular acupuncture points and meridians are required to address specific syndromes. Acupuncture points have precise anatomical locations, at which a needle should be inserted to effect the desired result.

⟐ The patient has blood stagnation, commonly due to accidents, sports injuries, etc., that needs to be released by needling or lancing the affected area.

⟐ The patient has symptoms that can be released by the use of motor or trigger points; often, deeper needling is required to release these muscle areas.

⟐ The patient is ungrounded and retention of acupuncture needles in the body will help to alleviate the situation.

Acupuncture Needles and Tuning Forks: A Powerful Synergy

The combined effect of treatment with acupuncture needles and tuning forks permits access both to Kidney essence and the Water element, and the electrical response of the body to the action of the acupuncture needle, which evokes aspects of the Fire element. Acu-sound points that represent a blending of these energies archetypally embody, vibrationally and electrically, attributes of the planets Venus and Mars.

Acupuncture Needles Are from Mars/ Tuning Forks Are from Venus

In our sound-healing seminars taught around the world in the past two decades, MichelAngelo would illustrate the difference between the two modalities by paraphrasing the title of John Gray's best-selling book about relationships,[4] by making the following analogy: "Acupuncture needles are from Mars, and tuning forks are from Venus." Each of these planetary archetypes describes a different mode of engagement with the body from a healing perspective.

The Needle: Mars

The needle itself, historically manufactured from iron, is a long, slender, phallic instrument, engineered to pierce the integument of the skin for a specific purpose. While original shamanic practices, predating the historical development of acupuncture, would have seen this action as providing an avenue for the release of malign spirits, in the modern era, needles retained in the skin stimulate the body's immune response. This enhances blood circulation and the flow of energy at the site of the insertion. Acupuncture needling is mildly invasive, and when taken into consideration with the other factors, it is regarded as Martian in thrust.

Tuning Forks: Venus

By way of contrast, tuning forks, as resonators and transmitters of targeted sound vibration, are carefully placed upon the body at designated acupuncture points, in the chakras or muscles, or introduced into the energy field, and are completely noninvasive. Healing sound engages the receptive human faculty of hearing, accomplished through the sound-gathering apparatus of the outer ear. As noted above, these vibrations, independent of actual processing of them by the cerebral cortex, can produce noteworthy effects at the cellular level. One of Venus' principal attributes is that of relationship, and the skillful practitioner of sound healing fosters a transitory vibratory rapport with the patient that is organic, gentle, and persistent in its effect beyond the mere application or perception of the sound itself.

Synergize both modalities in the following instances.

⬧ The patient has prenatal and/or postnatal Qi-related imbalances.

⬧ There are Kidney Qi and essence deficiencies as well as digestive issues.

⬧ Both Yin and Yang organs and meridians need balancing.

⬧ Tuning forks can balance, vibrate, and tone excess and deficiency imbalances simultaneously; the localized stimulation of acupuncture points with both needle insertions and vibration permits the practitioner to target specific constitutional imbalances. Due to the adaptogenic nature of sound vibration, the danger of overtreating is minimized, whereas, as we have indicated earlier, overtreatment in sessions using acupuncture needles occurs on a regular basis.

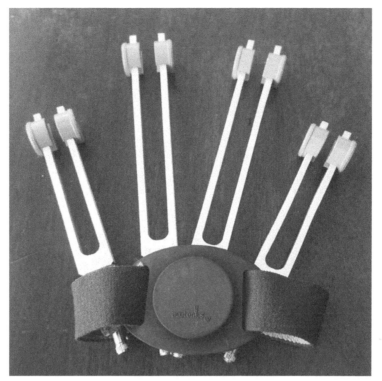

Figure 2.1 *Acutonics Ohm® tuning forks and belted acuvator*

Benefits and Contraindications of Sound Resonance
BENEFITS

⬧ Promotes the development of healthy sleep patterns.

⬧ Alleviates stress.

⬧ Lifts depression.

⬧ Positively impacts and balances blood pressure.

⬧ Reduces fever.

⬧ Ameliorates painful conditions.

⬧ Promotes memory retention and greater efficiency of learning.

⬧ The two sets of Acutonics Ohm® forks, referred to as the Acutonics Ohm® Unison and Low Ohm Unison, which we recommend in this book, root, ground, balance, and calm the Shen.

⬧ Noninvasive; good for needle-phobic patients.

- Tuning forks, because they do not penetrate the skin, do not cause bruising; consequently, they can be used to treat hemophiliacs or patients who are currently on regimes of blood-thinning medications.

- Tuning forks are safer for patients who have had plastic surgery.

- Tuning forks are effective in scar therapy treatments, anywhere on the face and body, for example, scars resulting from facelift surgery.

- Tuning forks can be used to treat patients who have pacemakers.

CONTRAINDICATIONS

- Do not use low-frequency tuning forks above the waist; this can cause the Yang to rise to the head and can contribute to a headache.

- All of the contradictions are similar to those of acupuncture, i.e., contraindicated points for needling/forking.

Benefits and Contraindications of Acupuncture Needling

Acupuncture addresses the entire body, face, and scalp, as do tuning fork treatments.

BENEFITS

The following conditions may be addressed with acupuncture.

- Dermatological issues such as acne, rosacea, eczema, etc. can be treated with topical/internal applications of Chinese herbs.

- Irregularities in the reproductive cycle and other gynecological imbalances.

- Sinus issues, headache, and other respiratory symptoms.

- Diarrhea, constipation, and a wide range of gastrointestinal issues.

- Thyroid problems; hyper- and hypothyroid conditions tend to manifest with the onset of menopause and can be treated with the Eight Extraordinary meridians (see Chapter 3), which address the endocrine system.

- Sensory organs—eyes, ears, nose, mouth—and brain imbalances.

- Insomnia, dizziness, vertigo, palpitations, mental/emotional imbalances, and general edema and puffiness of the face and body.

CONTRAINDICATIONS

- Do not treat hemophiliacs, because they bleed and bruise easily.

- Exercise caution in needling patients who have been prescribed blood-thinning medications; they are also subject to bleeding and bruising.

- Hypertension: make sure that the patient is taking their blood pressure medication. (See Chapter 7, and utilize the Fire element treatment for high blood pressure.)

- Be cautious in treating patients with diabetes; make certain that they are taking their medications. Diabetics are likewise prone to bruise and bleed.

- Avoid treating patients who have had a surgical facelift, Botox, or filler injections for a period of six months, until the effects of these procedures have worn off.

- If a patient has had laser resurfacing, microdermabrasion, or a chemical peel, you should wait for a period of two to six weeks prior to treating them with facial needling. The surface of the epidermis, the top layer of the skin, has been exfoliated. This leaves them vulnerable to infection.

- Use caution with patients who have chronic immune deficiency; "less is more" is better for these patients. (See "Metal Element" in Chapter 7 for treatment points that address immune deficiency.)

- Be careful in treating patients with chronic fatigue, and also those with adrenal deficiency. (See "Water Element" in Chapter 7.)

- Do not treat pregnant women with contraindicated points using acupuncture needles and/or Acutonics Ohm® Unison tuning forks. The following points will promote labor and are contraindicated:

- LI-4 Hegu, Joining Valley

- St-18 Rugen, Root of Breast (difficult labor)

- Bl-60 Kunlun, Kunlun Mountains

- Bl-67 Zhiyin, Reaching Yin (turns the fetus around, in cases of breech birth, and facilitates labor)

- GB-21 Jianjing, Shoulder Well (difficult labor, helps in the expulsion of the placenta).

Supplies Needed for Acu-Sound Treatments

Whether you choose to utilize only acupuncture needles or tuning forks, or to integrate both modalities, it is important to have the requisite supplies. For acupuncture treatments, I recommend using the Japanese Seirin needles; they are gentle, strong, and manufactured according to exacting specifications and rigorous standards. MichelAngelo and I had occasion to visit the Seirin factory in Shimizu, Japan, some years ago during a teaching trip, and it is quite apparent that they take great pains to produce superior-quality acupuncture needles. I strongly advise you to use Seirin needles that are packaged with guide tubes. You can easily insert them into the skin without causing your patient undue stress; the Japanese are not advocates of painful acupuncture needling, and this product reflects that aesthetic.

Acupuncture Needles

- Seirin red #1: 0.16 gauge, 30 mm

- Seirin red #1: 0.16 gauge, 15 mm

- Seirin ivory #2: 0.18 gauge, 30 mm

- Seirin blue #3: 0.20 gauge, 30 mm

- Seirin purple #5: 0.25 gauge, 40 mm

You will also need the following:

- Wan Hua oil or Arnica gel/cream for bruising.

❖ Arnica homeopathic pellets (6C for acute bruising/12C for chronic bruising).

❖ Two silver spoons, which are iced prior to the treatments and can be effectively used to disperse bruises. The simplest way to cool them down is to fill a cup with ice cubes and immerse the spoons in it until they are needed.

Tuning Forks

❖ 1 pair Acutonics Ohm® tuning forks, aka Ohm Unison set

❖ 1 pair Acutonics® Low Ohm tuning forks, aka Low Ohm Unison set

❖ 1 belted acuvator; we recommend this as more efficient than the alternate tabletop acuvator. The problem with the latter is that, unless you have a small table of the requisite height in your clinic, you will be compelled to place it on the treatment table. This is not a sufficiently firm surface for striking the acuvator; consequently, you will not achieve much in the way of vibrations when you strike the forks. Moreover, to hammer away upon the same table where your patient is lying would be disruptive for them, to say the least.

The belted acuvator is strapped around the thigh, and by striking the two forks successively, hand over hand, on the raised pad, you will be able to produce the desired resonances.

Let us offer some recommendations regarding best practices for tuning fork activation.

❖ First of all, while we naturally hear sound with our ears, it is the palpable waves produced by a resonating source, which subsequently travel through the atmosphere, that stimulate our hearing faculty. Those same waves engender a visceral experience, which is intensified by vibrations of higher amplitude; in other words, the more vibration that can be introduced by the application of a particular tuning fork combination, the more agreeable the effect to the patient, and the deeper into the body those vibrations penetrate. Therefore, your intention is to produce as much resonance as possible in the most efficient manner.

◈ There are two schools of thought as to how best to hold the tuning forks—by the stem or by the yoke. There are many skilled practitioners who advocate the former technique, and it might seem that such a grip would not impede the transmission of the vibrations of the fork's tines. However, when a tuning fork is resonating, the area between the tines, the yoke, is largely devoid of vibration as the tines oscillate back and forth. Therefore, the resonating frequency travels unencumbered past the yoke, through the stem, and into the body.

Additionally, the round stem of the tuning fork does not afford the practitioner a firm grasp upon the instrument, and the probability of dropping it by accident is correspondingly increased, whereas the flat surface of the yoke seems ideal for gripping between the pads of the thumb and forefinger.

◈ Striking the forks on the belted acuvator requires a certain coordination, and it is important to find a comfortable way to do so. Often, neophyte practitioners are extremely timid about using enough force to resonate the tuning forks, and consequently, very little vibration is felt by the patient.

While we would not wish to advocate the use of excessive force in a therapeutic context, it is important to strike the forks with sufficient vigor to produce a highly resonant result—one that will have a certain duration upon the body and impart the healing vibrations. I usually recommend that the practitioner thinks of them as hammers striking a nail, although there is one slight caveat to accompany this suggestion. Often, particularly with middle-frequency forks, which do not vibrate as readily as low-frequency ones, a vigorous impact of the flat surface of the colored resonator (the gold-colored disks that are positioned on the ends of the tines) on the acuvator produces an unwanted secondary sound—an audible clink. I have likened many Acutonics® seminars to blacksmiths' conventions because of the preponderance of this sound in the practicum sessions, although I rather suspect that, as we learned in Chapter 1, Pythagoras would not disapprove of that ambience! Once again, this clinking noise, particularly heard in close proximity to the head, would not be particularly restful for the patient. This can be avoided by simply striking a resonator of each tuning fork upon the acuvator on an *outside* edge.

There is also a learning curve with achieving similar resonance with both forks, as the majority of people are not ambidextrous, and they are a bit awkward with their less dominant hand. It takes practice.

◆ As to the activation of the forks themselves, I usually inform practitioners that there are two components, one Yang, one Yin.

- Yang: the strike itself; it should be made with straightforward vigor, with a loose, flexible wrist that permits you to deliver the impact without undue force.

- Yin: the release; often neophytes execute the strike with a stiff wrist, and there is no rebound. This immediately deadens the resulting tone. Allowing the forks to rebound naturally following the strike will maximize the resonance.

- We also suggest that the movements of the hands and arms should be smooth and fluid, as if the practitioner were executing the graceful postures of Tai Chi. It is recommended that the practitioner should maintain an upright stance when administering the vibrations, rather than bend to make contact with the acu-sound points on the face and body.

Treatment Length and Timeline

Please be aware that the integration of these two separately dynamic healing modalities will produce a cumulative effect that is powerfully transformational. We are merging and marrying Yin and Yang and harnessing the archetypal energy of the planets Venus, representing the feminine, and Mars, the embodiment of the masculine, qualities of receptivity and action, and additionally, the essence of the Metal and the Fire elements.

In an initial integrated treatment session of one hour, do not treat your patient for more than 25–35 minutes, which allows them the opportunity to rest and relax for the remainder of the 60 minutes. You will need to gauge how long it takes for them to receive the benefits of this synergetic approach. The use of the tuning forks as an adaptogen will provide further safeguard against overtreatment.

The tangible feedback provided to you by the gradually diminishing vibration of the tuning forks will alert you as to when your patient's body is no longer absorbing the resonance. Over time, you will undoubtedly find that your intuitive intelligence will notify you that this threshold has been reached. Feeling the vibrations creeping up your forearm indicates that it is you who is receiving the treatment, not the patient. Your patient is now thoroughly "cooked." You may put the tuning forks aside and, if you are using acupuncture needles, remove them from the body *prontissimo*. Venus checks Mars, and receptivity and harmony balance self-assertion and power.

Tuning Forks Only

The cultivation of vibratory relationship with your patient's body by means of tuning forks requires you to be receptive and grounded, tuning into your patient's energetic state. This state of heightened sensitivity is essential to this type of vibrational healing.

A session can range in length from 25 to 45 minutes, depending upon the needs of your patient; if you augment your vibratory arsenal with additional sound healing devices, for example, Tibetan or crystal singing bowls, tingsha, gongs, chimes, bells, etc., the session may last anywhere from 60 to 90 minutes.

See the Introduction for descriptions of these other sound tools and how you might employ them in your treatments.

Acupuncture Needling

Acupuncture, by itself, is a powerful and extraordinary healing modality that has a distinguished history of practice of more than 4000 years. As an acupuncturist of many years' standing and experience, I'm constantly reminded that one of my principal challenges is to know what points to needle and when to remove those needles so as not to overtax the patient. Overtreatment is a rather more common event in acupuncture sessions than in those involving tuning forks.

Conclusion

Vibrational Acupuncture™ is a cutting-edge holistic treatment approach that is unprecedented, one that blazes a new path in the complementary medicine field. It is an original synergy of two seemingly disparate transformational healing modalities, which will present you, the practitioner, with a multitude of new avenues for treating your patients, your loved ones, and yourself. In our experience, the vibrational approach works instantaneously, and it addresses disharmonies of body and spirit in a profound manner.

The integration of the diverse philosophical and theoretical approaches, ancient and modern, in this innovative modality—vibrational healing, acupuncture, Western astrological (planetary) medicine, Western and Chinese music theory, and Chinese medicine—grounds it in centuries of knowledge, wisdom, and rich tradition.

Chapter 3

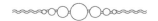

The Eight Extraordinary Meridians and Our Genetic Imprint

The body knows and remembers, while the mind only thinks it knows—and forgets.

Mary Elizabeth Wakefield

In this chapter, we introduce the first of our three levels of treatment: the Jing, or prenatal Qi, which is embodied in the Eight Extraordinary meridians. Even though much has been contributed to the literature on these important channels in recent years, there have been, in our experience, no treatment protocols advanced that address a synergy of tuning forks with acupuncture needling on these meridians.

The Eight Extraordinary vessels, as embodiments of prenatal Qi, represent DNA, or our genetic blueprint, and the physical traits that we inherit from our ancestors, such as the shape of our eyes, the color of our skin and hair, and our height, among other things. We also inherit qualities, specific talents, habits, health imbalances, addictive tendencies, and predispositions to psycho-emotional illnesses such as chronic depression. These tendencies are stored in our cellular memory and made manifest in our blood.

We will present some unique concepts and protocols, including the following.

⬥ Fascia Talk, the palpation of the fascia (connective tissue) to discern which master/couple points of the Eight Extraordinary meridians to use in a given treatment.

◈ Specific treatment protocols for these channels that utilize components of sacred geometry:

- the Earth planetary glyph

- the figure 8/infinity symbol

- the Sound Tube.

◈ In addition to physical indications for these meridians, we are also including some psychospiritual considerations that depart from the common archetypal associations of the Eight Extraordinary meridians found in standard textbooks on the subject.

The Eight Extraordinary meridians (Qi Jing Ba Mai) were identified for the first time in *The Yellow Emperor's Classic of Internal Medicine* (*Nei Jing*). It is difficult to translate the pictographs that delineate Chinese words into English, because these symbols can be interpreted in a variety of ways depending upon the context. In Chinese medicine, the words used to describe these channels represent both the meridians' functions and their individual identity. For example, the word "Qi" relates to the functional flow of energy in other meridians, for example, the Lung meridian. However, the Qi of the Eight Extraordinary meridians is unique and exceptional, belonging only to them. Therefore, multiple descriptive words were used to explain the special value of these channels.

Qi Jing Ba Mai

Qi: is something unusual, different, exceptional, strange, rare, wonderful, miraculous, as well as something extra, beyond the mundane aspect of existence. This Qi pertains to ancestral Qi, our genetic blueprint, the creation of life, and the birth of a child.

Jing: is the clearest distillation of genetic essence and is linked to the core of our individual identity. It is a channel, an enclosed tubular passageway, a conduit through which the natural ancestral waterway of Kidney essence flows.

Ba: represents the number eight, and specifically relates to longevity; it also evokes orientation in physical space, such as we find in the Bagua. The digit "8" is akin to the universal symbol for infinity.

Mai: this is the vessel itself, which is not only a pathway, but also a canal. It is likened to an artery that allows Jing to circulate throughout the body.[1]

It is important to note that the Eight Extraordinary vessels have specific attributes and properties that distinguish them from the Twelve Regular meridians:

⬩ They interact with the Twelve Regular meridians but do not have an internal/external organ relationship with them. However, they influence the internal organs.

⬩ While these channels have master/couple points, they do not have any points of their own, except for the Du Mai and Ren Mai.

⬩ They are conduits of prenatal Qi and are fueled by Kidney essence.

⬩ Their Qi does not move in one direction, but ebbs and flows like the tides.

⬩ And, very important, the names of the Eight Extraordinary meridians are indicative of their special function, as opposed to the Twelve Regular meridians, which represent postnatal Qi and relate to the organ systems and their energetic function.

Master/Couple Points of the Eight Extraordinary Meridians

While I am treating these channels with acupuncture needles and/or Acutonics Ohm® Unison tuning forks, I always begin with the master point in order to open the Qi of the meridian; then I follow with the couple point contralaterally.

However, the master point(s) that is customarily associated with each meridian is not always the opening/master point. For example, for Chong Mai, Sp-4 Gongsun may not be the master point; it could just as easily be PC-6 Neiguan, Inner Pass that is indicated as the master point that will open the energy of the Chong Mai.

Please read the guidelines regarding my system of Fascia Talk diagnostics in this chapter. This technique is an unusual way to test for, and discern, which master point should be addressed first in a treatment. Even if you are not an acupuncturist, this approach will be useful to you.

Master (Chong Mai): Penetrating Vessel

Sp-4 Gongsun, Grandfather/Grandson is located on the medial side of the foot, in the depression distal and interior to the first metatarsal bone. It regulates the Spleen Qi, resolves dampness, calms the Shen, and benefits the Heart and chest. It also treats depression and self-pity.

Couple (Yin Wei Mai): Yin Linking Vessel

PC-6 Neiguan, Inner Pass is on the flexor aspect of the forearm, 2 cun (inches) proximal to PC-7 Daling, between the tendons of the palmaris longus and flexor carpi radialis. This point opens the chest, regulates the Heart, and calms the Shen; it also alleviates nausea and clears heat. It can be used to treat people who have heart issues, who are frightened, and who have difficulty receiving from others.

Master (Ren Mai): The Conception Vessel

Lu-7 Lieque, Broken Sequence is on the radial aspect of the forearm, approximately 1.5 cun proximal to LI-5 Yangxi, in the cleft between the tendons of the brachioradialis and abductor pollicis longus. This point expels wind, releases the interior, descends Lung Qi, and breaks up phlegm. It also regulates the water passages and alleviates pain in the head and the nape of the neck. It is the command point for the head and the face. Psychospiritually, it can be used to help patients who are suffering from grief and sadness, and who are troubled by survival issues.

Couple (Yin Qiao Mai): Yin Heel Vessel

Kid-6 Zhaohai, Shining Sea is below the prominence of the medial malleolus in the groove formed by two ligamentous bundles. This point nourishes Yin, clears heat, benefits the eyes, and calms the spirit. It can be used to treat patients with difficult urination; it also benefits the throat and promotes self-esteem and self-confidence.

Master (Du Mai): Governing Vessel

SI-3 Houxi, Back Stream is located on the ulnar border of the hand, in the depression proximal to the head of the fifth metacarpal bone. SI-3 Houxi benefits the neck, the occiput, and the back; it alleviates pain, clears wind, helps with eye pain, and calms the Shen. It also clears the mind, providing a sense of clarity and the strength to face difficult decisions and life choices. Heat and wind in this channel can cause more serious conditions such as epilepsy and manic depression.

Couple (Yang Qiao Mai): Yang Heel Vessel

UB-62 Shenmai, Extending Vessel is on the lateral side of the foot, approximately 0.5 cun inferior to the inferior border of the lateral malleolus, in a depression posterior to the peroneal tendons. It extinguishes internal wind, treats epilepsy, benefits the head and legs, and alleviates pain. It calms the Shen and is effective in the treatment of mania, epilepsy, dizziness, and insomnia. This point represents our purpose and how we extend ourselves to the world.

Master (Dai Mai): Belt Vessel

GB-41 Zulinqi, Foot Governor of Tears is in the depression distal to the junction of the fourth and fifth metatarsal bones, on the lateral side of the tendon of the exterior digitorum longus muscle. It promotes the flow of Liver Qi, clears damp heat (such as in vaginal discharge), and treats migraines and eye disorders. It extinguishes internal wind and dissipates phlegm nodules. This point can empower a person who is fighting back their tears to express their anger and frustration.

Couple (Yang Wei Mai): Yang Linking Vessel

TH-5 Waiguan, Outer Pass is 2 cun proximal to TH-4 Yangchi in the depression between the radius and the ulna, on the radial side of the extensor digitorum communis tendon. This point releases the exterior, expels wind and heat, and subdues Liver Yang, such as is manifest in migraine headaches. It also alleviates pain, calms the Shen spirit, and helps a person to set appropriate boundaries in relationships.

Fascia Talk

The modern Western medical term *fascia* derives from a Latin noun meaning "bundle." Fascia—a sheet of connective tissue that is mostly collagen—stabilizes, surrounds, and separates muscles and internal organs.

Dr. Daniel Keown, M.B., Ch.B., Lic.Ac., quotes a passage from the *Nan Jing* in which the Triple Heater (Burner) is described as "the organ with a name, but no form":[2]

The Triple Heater (Burner) is also key to understanding acupuncture, since it is none other than the patterns created and modeled in the body by fascia. Fascia, a substance that has no form of its own, takes on the form of that which it is covering.[3]

According to Dr. Keown, acupuncture points are found between the spaces of the fascial layers. Fascia contains fibrous connective tissue packed in bundles of collagen fibers that are parallel to the direction of pull. Fascia is flexible and can tolerate considerable stress and unidirectional tension.

Fascia Facts

- Fibroblasts are the precursor to collagen/elastin production, and they are located in the fascia.

- Fascia is similar to ligaments and tendons due to their collagen content.

- Fascia differs in location and function.

- Fascia surrounds muscles and other structures.

Fascia Talk is an innovative diagnostic technique that permits the practitioner to discern which Eight Extraordinary meridian point is the master point and which is the couple.

The quote provided as the epigraph to this chapter is accurate; it describes the body's innate intelligence and its awareness of the inherited legacy of cellular memory, especially when it pertains to the Eight Extraordinary meridians.

"The Body Knows and Remembers…"

The body not only is a repository of memory, but can also instruct us as to which acupoints are needed for treatment and exactly where those points are to be located. Most of my patients will, at some time during their sessions, say to me, "No, that's not the point; it is here!" Without any training whatsoever, these patients demonstrate the ability to tune into the messages that their bodies are transmitting, making them aware of the flow of Qi and what points will best facilitate their healing process. I listen to them and find that, most of the time, they are right on the mark.

"...the Mind Only Thinks It Knows–and Forgets"

The second half of the quote is for the practitioner, friend, colleague, or family member who is using Fascia Talk as a diagnostic tool. As acupuncturists, having wielded our diagnostic skills—tongue, pulse, hara, the Four Exams—we feel certain that we know which master point should be needled first and which Eight Extraordinary meridians will address the patient's constitutional imbalances.

As a result of my many years of clinical practice, I cannot help but think that my assessment of the patient's condition is accurate; nevertheless, the simple truth is that I am not always right. Our bodies are incapable of lying. The mind should not be the only faculty engaged when you are working with the soma. A primal understanding of what is needed, based upon one's perception of the information coded in the patient's cellular memory, takes over.

While I will be introducing a protocol for assessing the body's needs via my system of Fascia Talk, there are other somatic diagnostic testing methods with which some of you may be familiar.

- Body Talk: in this system, the practitioner employs neuromuscular feedback, intuition, and balancing techniques using hand positions and light tapping on the heart. Apparently, the tapping causes an interruption of the energy connection between the brain and the heart, disrupting preexisting dysfunctional programming. As a result, it can encourage the patient to adopt new modes of behavior and effect beneficial change in their life.

- Applied kinesiology (muscle testing): this technique claims to discover health imbalances by testing the strength vs. weakness of muscles or muscle groups. In a manual muscle test, the patient raises their arm and resists the downward applied force of the practitioner, while questions are being asked about whether a nutritional supplement is good for the body. The difference in muscle response can indicate the presence of various stressors or constitutional imbalances.

⬧ Japanese O-ring testing (BDORT): O-ring testing, invented by Yoshiaki Omura, is similar to applied kinesiology. The patient forms an "O" with their thumb and index finger, and the practitioner tests their strength by trying to pry the two digits apart, while the patient holds a sample medication or potential allergen in their free hand. This test, apparently, can assess the patient's health and need for treatment.

Guidelines for Fascia Talk Diagnostics

The simplest way to engage with your patient's body is to seek a straightforward answer—either "yes" or "no." You can then use these responses to ascertain which master point on which meridian should be treated.

1. First, ask your patient for permission to touch (palpate) their thigh or upper arm. Explain to them that this is for diagnostic purposes.

2. Place one hand on the patient's thigh or their upper arm (there is a great deal of fascia in the thighs).

3. Program their body to provide a "yes" or "no" response; I usually move the fascia upward toward the head for "yes" and downward toward the feet for "no."

4. Make sure that the fascia moves easily. If the fascia doesn't move easily, it is tight and needs to be gently moved up and down until it releases. Sometimes the patient will be wearing leggings or tight jeans. The patient should change into more loose-fitting pants.

5. Having established the dynamics of the fascial response, you will not need to physically move it again. You can reinforce the programming by asking the patient a series of simple questions that require a yes or no answer and sensing the result through the movement of the fascia in the appropriate direction. Note that this will not be a gross upward or downward movement, but rather more of a gentle floating in either direction; it is quite subtle.

6. In order to conduct the diagnostics, I hold one hand in position on the thigh or upper arm and, using my free hand, point to the specific Eight Extraordinary meridian point that has been

indicated by my other diagnostic approaches—tongue, pulse, hara palpation, etc.

7. For example, if I have ascertained that the patient has an imbalance in the Ren Mai, I will point to Lu-7 Lieque. If the fascia should move downward under my other hand, that is a resounding "no." I will then test the other point on the Ren Mai, Kid-6 Zhaohai, on the medial ankle bone.

8. If the fascia then moves upward, which indicates "yes," I will regard Kid-6 Zhaohai as my master point, and needle or fork it first. I will then follow with the couple point Lu-7 Lieque, on the thumb side of the wrist.

Should Ren Mai not be indicated in this process, I will test the master points for the other Eight Extraordinary meridians—Chong Mai, Dai Mai, and Du Mai.

Trust is important in this process, as is being willing to heed the feedback provided by your patient's body. Sometimes I instruct students to close their eyes, because they are so used to relying upon them as part of their diagnostic skills; if they are excessively visual, they won't feel anything.

I find that this approach to working with the prenatal Qi is very effective, and receptivity is essential to this kind of diagnostic skill. Temporarily disconnecting the brain from its visual input, the capacity to listen—the less-valued intuitive faculty—is brought to the fore, and the sense of touch is correspondingly heightened. I remind my students about the blind *ammas* in Japan, whose every finger functions like a little "ear."

Sacred Geometry Treatments for the Eight Extraordinary Meridians
Guidelines

◈ Treat only one set of the Eight Extraordinary meridians, contralaterally. Do not overtreat.

◈ Needle the master point first and then the couple point. Utilize the Acutonics Ohm® Unison tuning forks to draw the sacred geometry symbols *around* the needles three times.

⁕ You can also use the tuning forks by themselves on the master/ couple points, placing one fork on the point and then using the other to sketch the appropriate symbol (three times).

Recommended Treatments

THE PLANETARY GLYPH OF EARTH: THE CROSS ⊕

In Chapter 1, we introduced the planetary glyph for Earth, which is a cross, or two intersecting lines, sometimes referred to as the cross of time and space. In an era in which most of us have regular recourse to global positioning systems, a cross establishes a grid of latitude and longitude upon the surface of the Earth, which allows us to position ourselves at a precise location.

A cross is similarly a meeting point, a location where individuals can encounter people with whom they are not familiar and consequently be exposed to new ideas. The horizontal axis of the cross is like two arms that have the capacity to embrace or reject a loved one or accept or reject creative input. The lines of a cross flow toward the center; this is illustrative of the inexorable and inescapable gravitational pull exerted upon us by Earth. We are only freed of the burden of our weight here on Earth when we surrender our bodies at the end of life to continue our souls' journeys. The four quadrants delineated by the cross are also representative of the energy of manifestation, which is only possible when we are supported by a vital Earth connection.

TREATMENT: EARTH GLYPH

1. Needle the master/couple points contralaterally, then vibrate the Acutonics Ohm® Unison tuning forks, inscribing the Earth glyph, the cross, upon the body and/or above it, three times.

2. You can also employ tuning forks only to draw the Earth glyph upon or above the body.

This treatment, with its additional emphasis upon Earth, in the form of the glyph, is very grounding. It helps your patient to establish themselves in present time and supports the manifestation of their creative goals in life.

The Figure 8/Infinity Symbol/Lemniscate
The Infinity Symbol ∞

In needling the master/couple points contralaterally, i.e., on the opposite side, an infinity symbol, a sacred geometry pattern, is created on your patient's body. For example, by first needling Du Mai SI-3 Houxi, Back Stream as the master point on the right side and the couple point Yang Qiao Mai Bl-62 Shenmei Extending Vessel on the left, and by viewing the patient's navel as the center of a figure-8 configuration, the other half of the symbol is energetically completed by the patient's own Qi on the other side of the body.

This completed energetic circuit is specifically related to ancestral Qi and the genetic blueprint of the patient. The number eight has a particular significance in Chinese numerology and is considered to relate to longevity. In general, by itself, we can view a figure 8 as a geometric configuration that has no beginning and no end; hence, it is infinite. Once again, it relates to the alchemical pursuit of immortality.

However, if we lay a figure 8 on its side, ∞, it becomes a specialized mathematical symbol known as the lemniscate, which is commonly used to designate infinity. The lemniscate is frequently utilized in esoteric iconography to indicate a certain numinosity, the idea being that the person or thing adorned with it possesses spiritual power and transcendence. Usage of a similar figure has been found in Tibetan rock carvings, and the antecedents of the symbol itself date back to ancient Greece. Some sources suggest that it is analogous to the final letter of the Greek alphabet, omega. It is often compared, as well, to the ancient image of the uroboros, a snake devouring its tail, which has considerable significance in alchemical tradition and is a potent symbol of death and rebirth. Thus, the invocation of the lemniscate pattern through this contralateral needling of the Eight Extraordinary meridians is powerfully resonant and transformative.

The fact that a patient's body will follow through energetically with the completion of the figure 8 on the side of the body that was not needled is a testimony to the intelligence of the human organism and the natural flow of Qi, which self-heals and self-harmonizes. This is why I do not recommend needling both sides of the body, except in rare circumstances, such as injuries on both sides of the body, an imbalance of Yin and Yang Qiao, and a corresponding imbalance between the right and left sides of the body, or if there is an indication for bilateral needling in the diagnostics.

Treatment: The Figure 8/Infinity Symbol

1. Needle the master/couple points.

2. Activate the Acutonics Ohm® Unison tuning fork combination and inscribe the infinity symbol three times on, or above, the body, around the needle three times.

3. Use the head of the needle as the omphalos, i.e., the center, of the figure 8.

4. You can use the Acutonics Ohm® Unison tuning forks by themselves; vibrate them around the implied master point, followed by the couple point, three times, focusing the energy of the figure 8 symbol.

Treatment: The Sound Tube

Some years ago, Acutonics® and I collaborated on creating faceted gem tips that could be attached to the stem of their Ohm tuning forks. After several years of research and development, a superb bored-out version of their basic Ohm forks, with an engineered screw-on cap, was perfected. This fork can be used as is, or the cap may be removed and any number of individual gem tips may then be screwed onto the Ohm tuning forks.

In working with these unique vibratory tools, I became fascinated with the hollow tube in the base of the new bored-out Ohm forks. This encouraged me to begin experimenting with the idea of resonating this vibratory tube over an acupuncture needle. I also tested various metals, such as stainless steel, gold, silver, and copper, to see if they responded differently to the vibrations imparted to them by the tube. The results were as follows.

- Stainless steel needles balance the patient.

- Gold needles tonify adrenal deficiency, boost immunity, and address general psychospiritual imbalances.

❖ Silver needles disperse any excess patterns, for example, excess phlegm in the chest cavity, too much heat, a wiry Liver, which manifests as irritability and frustration, etc.

❖ Copper needles are perfect conductors and accentuate the vibration of the tuning forks, which then travels to wherever it may be needed.

- We can correlate this remarkable conductivity with copper's ancient associations with Aphrodite and the planet Venus; according to myth, the Mediterranean island of Cyprus was where Aphrodite first made landfall, in an area that was historically rich in copper deposits. This led to the metal being designated by the Greeks as *cyprium*, which became the Latin *cuprum*, and hence, copper.

- In medieval manuscripts, the same symbol is used for both the planet Venus and copper (♀).

- This conductivity is related to two factors that can be seen as related to archetypal Venus; the first is the metal's softness at room temperature. This can be likened to a yielding, Venusian quality, more Yin than Yang.

- The second has to do with the fact that only a single electron inhabits the outer shell of the copper atom. Thus, copper can more readily lend itself to vibratory relationship through electron exchange with other atoms. On a practical level, this translates into extreme conductivity, as electrons can pass easily from one copper atom to another, with very little resistance.[4]

1. Needle the master and couple point.

2. Use two bored-out Ohms as sound tubes and insert them over the needles.

3. You can treat both master and couple points simultaneously, three times.

Psychospiritual Interpretations of the Eight Extraordinary Meridians

As part of the educational mission of *Chi-Akra Center for Ageless Aging*, we have created a myriad of seminars over the past 20 years, the majority of which focus on the transformation of the facial landscape. However, consistent with Mary Elizabeth's constitutional approach to this modality, as espoused in her book *Constitutional Facial Acupuncture*, a firm constitutional grounding to the various facial protocols is always a part of the curriculum, of which material on the Eight Extraordinary channels is of the highest priority. Consequently, I have had ample opportunity to consider the symbolism and significance of the Eight Extraordinary meridians from a psychospiritual perspective, beyond the standard associations that are offered in textbooks on the subject. In our seminars, from extrapolations upon these archetypal considerations, I have offered my own personal interpretations of the extraordinarily potent terrain of these exceptional energy conduits.

Embryological Order

In the beginning, as we understand it from both science and myth, life originates from an amorphous, primeval, creative matrix. The Chinese refer to this as "no form"—the void, nothingness, Oneness, the Great One, designated as the Tai Ye, the Yin/Yang symbol, in Taoist philosophy.

The One, unmanifest potentiality, over vast eons of time, eventually fissions itself into two distinct and complementary forces, the Yin/Yang, female/male, *et al.* The evolution of these primal polarities establishes the foundation for the evolution of higher life-forms through successive differentiation into structures of increasing complexity, a process that is mirrored in the development of the fetus in the womb from an insignificant blob of protoplasm to a fully formed infant.

This dual expression of Yin and Yang facilitates our emergence as human organisms into physical being. The divine, perfect in its unanimity, nevertheless seeks greater knowledge of itself through manifestation into the seeming contrarieties of material existence. In the psycho-energetic paradigm of morphology that is described by the Eight Extraordinary meridians, we find a similar architecture of polarities. These primordial energetic conduits arise in pairs, with the exception of Chong Mai, which represents the untrammeled flow of genetic inheritance as it is transmitted from generation to generation—it is our blood, our tribe, our family ties.

Chong Mai

The Chong Mai, or Penetrating Vessel, is the first meridian to arise in the embryological order. It represents the moving Qi between the Kidneys and prenatal Jing, because the Chong relates to blood and is representative of our genetic heritage. It pinpoints a specific stream of humanity or consciousness in which we participate. This meridian, as the creative offspring of the Ren and Du channels, is an analogue of each of us as our parents' children.

All the other meridians arise from the Chong Mai, considered the most ancient of the Eight Extraordinary meridians. As it has its wellsprings deep within the body, between the Kidneys, and then courses through the interior organs of generation, i.e., Uterus and Prostate), it hearkens back to an earlier evolutionary state. We should note that Chong Mai encounters both the Ren (at the point of its issuance from the body) and later the Du (at the triple confluence of meridians that occurs at the upper lip), reinforcing its relationship with both.

The idea of genetic or familial inheritance connected with this channel is powerfully resonant. Throughout human history, bloodlines have transmitted the wealth of inheritance, forged alliances between disparate peoples, and determined the status of individuals within societies.

Picture this influence of the Chong Mai as a powerful torrent of memory flowing from past to present, erupting from the hidden realm of the collective unconscious within the recesses of the body, to find expression at the moment of our conception (Ren), and later refinement through the manifestation of our individual destiny (Du).

Chong Mai represents the surge of life that occurs at that pivotal moment when the twin polarities unite, as a spark of divine life descends from the heavens to enliven the infant *in utero.* Scientists have conclusively demonstrated in recent years that the first contact of sperm with egg evokes a flash of blue light, caused by a release of zinc;[5] this is like the lightning flash of Uranus the sky god fertilizing Mother Earth—captured in a single instant of supercharged creative fusion.

Interpersonal dynamics—and patterns of behavior, both constructive and destructive—are often recapitulated from generation to generation. Skeletons hidden within the family armoire will often include trauma—psychological, physical, or sexual. Even those individuals who have consciously divorced themselves from the family milieu may yet fall prey to these unconscious pitfalls. Consequently, they may seek release in all sorts of addictive behaviors to escape from the psychic burden of this subconscious memory.

The personalized spiritual pilgrimage involved in the itinerary of the Chong Mai has its origins in the underworld, deep within the recesses of the body, in the energetic terrain of the sexual chakra. This river of remembrance initially serves as a repository for the family shadow. Nevertheless, it should be noted that the river ascends steadily toward the higher chakras and the godhead. Continuing its upward trajectory, it forks and unites with the Kidney channels as they parallel the midline of the chest, traversing the transformational spiritual landscape of those acupuncture points on the chest and neck called the Kidney Spirit points and Windows of the Sky points. In entering the throat chakra, it becomes possible for these individuals to bring into consciousness the unspoken and forgotten transgressions, transcending the dysfunction that may be part of the warp and weft of their family's personal chronology, embedded in their cellular memory.

Ren Mai and Du Mai

This meridian pair represent the vertical axis of being and the energetic duality of front-and-back Qi movement. The first meridians to be formed, they contain the Mu and Shu points, the front and back chakras (in the Ayurvedic system), and the Taoist microcosmic orbit.

Ren Mai

In categorizing the Ren meridian as Yin, we can recognize that it represents a vehicle for receptivity. It presents to us, in large part, the principal interface between ourselves and our immediate environment, containing those sensory receptors—eyes, ears, nose, and mouth—through which we perceive the nature of material reality. It also houses those physical apparatuses through which we absorb the necessary substances—oxygen, food, light—that sustain our continued existence. Additionally, it contains within its terrain those anatomical features that are most readily linked to our notions of identity: our facial features and the external components of our sexual organs. It is the more vulnerable hemisphere of the body, in that our viscera lie just below the surface of the abdomen.

Ren Mai is traditionally labeled the Conception Vessel, which acknowledges its path traversing the entire central area between the groin and the throat. In all sexes, it connects the organs of reproductive generation and self-expression, and thus encompasses what we could refer to as the creative/procreative duality. This meridian's energetic trajectory thus echoes a fundamental precept of Hindu mysticism, in which these two areas of the body, associated with the second and fifth chakras, are in sympathetic resonance.

Dr. Leonard Shlain, in his book, *Sex, Time and Power*,[6] reports on a fascinating and explicit demonstration of this esoteric energetic linkage between the sexual organs and the throat. A certain species of male deer is mute except during that brief season of the year when it comes into rut. At that time, the increased flow of male hormones gives rise to an unprecedented phenomenon—the buck finds his hitherto elusive voice. He bellows forth his mating call, fiercely stimulated by the dictates of evolutionary need, and as the larynx descends into that unfamiliar territory within the throat, the buck's penis simultaneously thrusts forward. The redirected and rechanneled libido energy that finds its outlet through the throat is a distinctive signifier of sexual availability and potency.

Like that amorous ungulate, human beings are evolutionarily programmed to pursue the perpetuation of their genetic identity through the fostering of a new generation. This procreative imperative lies at the core of our being and drives us, in our discrete sexual identities, to seek the dissolution of the ego in union with the other.

The uterus may be regarded as an alchemical crucible in which the twin polarities of Yin and Yang merge to engender new life, securing the survival of not only our individual genome but also that of the species. It likewise represents the portal through which we enter into physical reality.

While we emerge from the womb fully formed in our corporeal nature, we cannot, at this stage in our life, be regarded as significantly different from the myriad other creatures that inhabit our planet. Possessing the organic equipment for communication, we are as yet incapable of spanning the distances that separate us from others except through physical means or rudimentary utterances lacking any linguistic significance. Such a quantum evolutionary leap only becomes self-evident after the development of individual consciousness, in which the Yin and Yang forces combine themselves yet again in the creative interplay of ideas between the twin hemispheres of the brain. Our ability to impart the concepts that characterize our unique identity is ultimately rendered manifest through speech. It is by means of this miraculous faculty, an essentially human attribute, that we fully claim our birthright.

The idea of birth, physical or creative, is thus crucial to an understanding of the Ren meridian. If we further examine the placement of this channel, we can see that in its positioning on the front of the body, it relates profoundly to the most intimate experiences of our lives. The oral/genital poles of the Ren are intrinsic to the procreative act that provides the stimulus for reproduction and are ultimately tied into our first physical relationship, that with our birth mother.

Mother is the predominant star in our neonatal cosmos and, in suckling us at her bosom, furnishing the vital sustenance we crave, she reinforces this most fundamental aspect of our Yin nature. The essential quality of receptivity is thus fostered through this loving embrace, Ren to Ren, and ideally she imparts to us not only lifegiving nourishment, but also warmth, protection, and security.

We drink in these psychospiritual nutrients with our mother's breast milk, absorbing them within our frail, developing psyches. This mirroring of our nascent humanity provides the springboard for the nurturance of a healthy ego structure, allowing us, in time, to form our own network of supportive relationships, starting with those in our family unit and expanding to include the greater community of which we are a part. Ultimately, the emergence of our sexual maturity leads inexorably to the desire for erotic fulfillment through intimate congress with the other, and the cycle begins anew.

In conjunction with the above, I have come to identify a key attribute of this particular meridian: vulnerability. Ren is the channel that seems most aligned to all those characteristics that define us as singular beings: our organs of perception, our external genitalia, our facial features, with their particular manifestations—eye and hair color, the shape of our faces, and the components of their individual physiognomy. Thus, in the pursuit of relationship, it is through the revelation of this ventral side of the body that we seek to attract the other.

We do not meet our intimate partners by provocatively rubbing our backsides together, however much some of us might enjoy that. We open our arms, physically and metaphorically, and expose/reveal ourselves. It is only in complete surrender to that potential for meaningful connection (and implicitly, physical, even mortal wounding) that we cultivate those circumstances under which it might occur. To behave otherwise, out of reticence or fear of rejection, short-circuits the process. Only in our capacity to be vulnerable to the other can we sow the seeds that may blossom into authentic relationship, one that transcends the relentlessly instinctual drive to foster offspring which will ensure our comparative immortality.

Du Mai

The Du Mai, or Governing Vessel, represents the manifestation or grounding of the creative potential of the Ren. In contrast to its partner, the Du traverses the Yang side, ascending from the perineum via the spine, over the top of the head, and terminating in the philtrum of the upper lip. Here, it flows both internally and externally into the Ren, completing what is known as the microcosmic orbit. The confluence of Ren and Du restores the ancient harmony of the primordial cosmic union and provides a vivid illustration of the cyclical nature of being, a symbolism embodied most memorably in the alchemical figure of the uroboros, a snake biting its own tail.

This anatomical progress from Yin to Yang reenacts the journey of creativity in both its cosmic and individual expressions, from conception (uterus) to manifestation (perineum). In a traditional Taoist meditation, the "water wheel," this energetic migration between the polarities takes place along the circumference of the microcosmic orbit. The practitioner directs the movement of breath accordingly, initiating the cycle of breath at the base of the spine at the origin of the Du meridian, allowing it to traverse the entire length of the combined trajectory of Du and Ren, ascending the back, and then descending the front of the body.

The Yang nature of the Du meridian may not be readily apparent in human beings, members of the warm-blooded, soft-skinned family *Mammalia*, but if we examine other taxonomic phyla, we can observe that the dorsal anatomy customarily incorporates any kind of protective integument, fins, scales, etc. Thus, the back is, by definition, the more armored component of the body, the spine itself our endogenous armature.

In light of the above, a keyword for Du Mai is *protection*. We human beings, thanks to the misguided efforts of the Titans Prometheus and Epimetheus—who failed to hold in reserve something of a protective nature for their prize creation, man, assigning such evolutionary advantages willy-nilly to other species—lack any such armoring against forces in the environment that might do us harm. Nevertheless, the spine, lying close as it does to the surface of the back, can be viewed as fulfilling this function. It is our backs that we present to others when they attack us emotionally—or to those with whom we are less than comfortable or who have, in some way, violated our sense of self. In extreme instances, we curl in upon ourselves to protect the delicate viscera that lie close to the surface of the ventral side of the body.

The spine is likewise the bulwark of our somewhat precarious bipedal stance (at least from an evolutionary perspective). Without it, like a circus tent without a central pole, we would collapse into a quivering mass of skin and soft tissue. It connects us both to Heaven and Earth, anchoring us in the realm of materiality but permitting us to reach for the stars.

While the Ren meridian is characterized by dependence and a desire for nurturance, the Du points us to those initial struggles for independence. In the same way that "ontogeny recapitulates phylogeny," according to zoologist Ernst Haeckel, the ongoing growth of human infants can be seen to mirror the developmental challenges encountered by the entirety of our species. The adorable baby, crawling about on all fours, bumping into all sorts of obstacles, is our primordial quadruped ancestor who, driven by the imperatives of natural selection, at some crucial juncture suddenly reared itself up on its hind legs.

When this occurs in those early stages of growth, the now-toddler begins to take their first decisive, albeit wobbly, steps away from Mother, who has hitherto comprised the entire ambit of their world, the source of all goodness. The drives of personal self-determination eventually overcome the recidivistic desire to cling to Mommy, to continue to derive comfort from those womblike feelings of security and safety. The child proceeds to embark upon their own journey of individual destiny, becoming the ultimate arbiter of their own fate.

The Du meridian mediates all significant transitions that we undergo during our maturation. It is often the case that we experience the trepidations associated with these necessary changes at the base of the spine, in the sacrum, from which, according to ancient wisdom, the

Eight Extraordinary meridians originally sprang. This "sacral blowout" might be likened to the fire of transformation burning at the core of our being, one that will not permit us to rest comfortably in the status quo and requires us to take necessary risks for our further prosperity and personal fulfillment.

Without the vital connection to Earth symbolized by the Du meridian, the individual has difficulty grounding their creative vision of themselves in any dynamic or enduring sense. They remain disconnected from the Source and prone to all sorts of insecurity concerning their continued well-being.

We suffer the loss of our Earth connection on an almost daily basis, cocooned (as many of us are) in our little domiciles of concrete, steel, and glass, far from the nurturing touch of the natural world. Much of our culture derives its technological sophistication from our harnessing of the Uranian energy of lightning, via the manipulation of the insubstantial, aerial agencies of electricity, and our immersion in the by-products of this electronic wizardry further "un-earths" us.

It was in this manner that the Greek hero Hercules was able to defeat one of his mythical nemeses, Tantalus, the son of Earth Mother Gaea, who drew his strength from contact with her. By holding his adversary helpless in the air, Hercules deprived Tantalus of life force and eventually overcame his much more physically impressive foe. In our fervent, unreasoning embrace of these new technologies, we have unwittingly positioned ourselves as the heirs of Tantalus. Our loss of Earth connection may ultimately prove to be our undoing as a species.

Dai Mai

The Dai Mai, or Belt meridian, represents the horizontal axis of the body and, with the vertical axes of the Du and Ren, forms the first four cells of a human embryo during the initial developmental phase of cellular mitosis.

The terrain of the Dai Mai, in contrast to the Chong Mai, might be likened to the personal rather than the familial shadow, those disowned, dishonored aspects of the personality that an individual may have suppressed in response to the conditioning of their family group, societal milieu, socio-economic status, etc. Reexamining this from the perspective of the Hindu chakra system, this vessel, which engirdles the waist, divides the seven principal chakras at the level of the solar plexus. The chakras that comprise the lower portion include the root, sexual, and solar plexus; the upper chakras are the heart, throat, third eye, and crown.

From the standpoint of personal evolution, the psychospiritual landscape of the three lower chakras tends to be more problematic than those of the other four. Fundamental drives such as those for survival and grounding (root), sexuality (sexual), and personal power (solar plexus) are those most likely to be impacted by external negative conditioning. Our discomfort with these aspects of ourselves, as we have grown to understand them through our contact with others, especially our family of origin, is a powerful stimulus for us to consign them to the nether regions of the unconscious.

We might further regard this corporeal division as being indicative of the duality of human existence. We are engaged in a perpetual struggle to tame the primal motivations and emotions embodied in the lower chakras, to transcend our insecurity, fear, and anger, harnessing them in the pursuit of our dreams, striving to more fully actualize our compassion, clarity, insight, and spiritual essence. As all-too-frail protoplasmic receptacles for the spark of divinity contained in our souls, we must recognize that the body itself is the shadow. However, while it may constrain us in our longing to embrace the Infinite, it nevertheless provides the vehicle whereby we may experience the sensuous splendors of the natural world and the authentic nature of our humanity.

The impact of such a perceived dichotomy between the mundane realm of matter and the "lofty" domain of spirit upon the human condition cannot be overestimated. A goodly portion of the history of Western civilization has been categorized by titanic conflicts between one religious group and another. This has certainly been the case in the last several decades of the modern era. The three Abrahamic religions—Judaism, Christianity, and Islam—are equally strident in their condemnation of the physical body as being the source of humanity's suffering.

The New Age is similarly polarized in its pursuit of spiritual verities at the expense of the health and well-being of the physical body and the recognition of the manifold blessings of incarnation. This movement has attracted multitudes of individuals who manifest this profound schism. There is a particular pathology in the desire to transcend the physical body by any means possible, and these persons are customarily unconscious due to their unwillingness to address the emotional toxicity trapped in their lower chakras and integrate those disowned aspects of themselves.

We are now witnessing parallel tendencies in those adherents of advanced technologies who advocate the abandonment of the burdens of corporeal existence for eternal life as a disembodied consciousness in a cybernetic organism. Our single-minded immersion in our increasingly omnipresent communications technology is likewise leaching the vitality from us as physical beings, robbing us of an essential aspect of our humanity, dimming our emotional intelligence, and sundering us from each other in ways that we have yet to assess.

If we choose to categorize these warring tendencies within ourselves as "light" and "darkness," we must acknowledge that one cannot exist without the other. Taking an example from nature, how much more transcendent the splendor of sunrise if we have eagerly anticipated it during the seeming endless blackout of a night without the comfort of the Moon? This seemingly ordinary event reenacts for us daily the creation of the universe, as the world is reborn out of darkness. This miraculous occurrence parallels the similar emergence of higher consciousness from the Stygian realm of the merely instinctual.

The Swiss founder of analytical psychology, Carl Jung, recognized the crucial importance of the integration of suppressed aspects of the personality—those consigned to an undeserved oblivion due to the censure of social and familial conditioning—as a necessary precursor to the development of the authentic Self. Through what we could describe as psychological alchemy, the Jungian analyst, together with their patient, labors to refine this *prima materia*, the raw, unredeemed essence of individual existence. Jung maintained that there was "gold" to be found within the obscurities of the shadow. Similarly, through a process of inner alchemy called "Nei-dan," Taoist mystics sought to transform the baser attributes of their being until they achieved their incorruptible "gold" nature. This involved not only the transformation of their spirit essence, or Shen, but also ultimately the physical body.

Qiao Vessels

The Qiao vessels are meridians that originate on the inside and outside of the heels and figure prominently in the individual's quality of engagement with the wider world, the manner in which they portray themselves within their environment. Each Qiao vessel employs a specific strategy for coping with life.

Yang Qiao Mai

As a Yang vessel, Yang Qiao is about further manifestations of self-assertion, moving beyond the assumption of the upright stance of independence embodied in the Du. The heels are the point of initial contact with the ground beneath us, and thus the quality of each of these meridians can be seen as a product of the individual's perception of their position within the world.

In its desire for self-expression, Yang Qiao pits itself against its environment in an adversarial manner, and in confronting impediments to its desires, seeks to blame circumstances beyond its control for those problems. These are individuals who inhabit a hostile universe and who remain blissfully unconscious of their own shortcomings as they confront the challenges of development. We might argue that the characteristic eversion of the feet associated with Yang Qiao opens the legs in such a way that the genitalia are displayed to all and sundry. This is a somewhat aggressive stance.

Yang Qiao types are the Type A personalities, activists in both the best and worst sense—those who are out to change the world. Their attitude is fundamentally one of resentment of the status quo, and they rebel against strictures that they feel will prevent them from manifesting their goals, no matter how self-serving they might be.

Yin Qiao Mai

Yin Qiao is rather more reticent about confrontation, with the Yin aspect of the channel traditionally associated with meditation. If we view Yang Qiao as relating to the active role of portrayal in the individual drama of one's life, then—resorting to the parlance of the theater—Yin Qiao is about the more subtle inner motivations that impel those choices of outer expression.

A crucial difference is the reaction to outer hindrances that deter the individual's manifestation of their desires. While Yang Qiao would prefer to simply bulldoze over any obstacle, Yin Qiao's default setting is to question its own sense of self-worth and to retreat rather than confront. Because of their intense inner life, they possess the capacity to reassess, reformulate, and attack the challenge anew. They may find greater illumination because they have the courage to question their entitlement, and the redoubling of their efforts, following a period of self-reflection, may indeed permit them to achieve the hitherto elusive end result. These are individuals who will seek assistance from others, but will also research solutions to problems themselves. This is a path of potentially greater consciousness than their resolutely outer-directed Yang Qiao counterpart.

The characteristically inverted foot position of Yin Qiao often requires corrective measures such as orthopedic shoes. It could also impede athletic endeavors and overall forward progress because of the awkwardness of the stance. The corresponding closed stance of the legs reflects the characteristically reserved nature of these types.

Wei Vessels

The two Wei meridians function as linking vessels that connect the inner (Yin) and outer (Yang) aspects of Qi movement. The separation of these twin aspects of ourselves permits us to experience life's lessons and is likewise necessary for incarnation into form. As we further conceptualize this idea of inner vs. outer, we can see that the distinction establishes recognizable parameters for physical existence. In the human body, the outer membrane of the skin serves as a critical boundary, the frontier between the self-contained integrity of our anatomy and the potentially harmful influences and forces in the environment. These two meridians represent a departure from the unity symbolized by the Tai Ye. Energetically, they relate to individualized desires and ambitions that may cause us to stray from the path of the Tao, distracting us from the pursuit of the fundamental harmony that may be achieved by an alignment with higher purpose.

Yin Wei Mai

Within the psychospiritual terrain associated with aging, we must recognize that the transmutation of Yang into Yin (and vice versa) inevitably forms a principal component of the ongoing maturation of human beings. We incarnate into physical form as demonstrably Yin, dependent upon others, especially our birth parents, for survival and satisfaction of our basic needs. During the secondary phase of our development, we gradually become more Yang, increasingly independent and self-reliant, seeking to establish our unique mark upon the world.

However, as we enter our fourth decade of existence (approximately), the marvelously self-renewing mechanisms that sustained an optimum level of metabolic functioning gradually ease out of overdrive. We embark upon what is normally perceived as an inexorable process of physical decline, which has as its ultimate destination the cessation of life.

The challenge of authentic maturation lies, therefore, in the ability to accommodate ourselves to the nature of this "devolution" from Yang to Yin. This is particularly challenging for those of us who live in the West because we are extraordinarily attached to our ego structures. Collectively, we have been conditioned by the Darwinist philosophy of "survival of the fittest" to regard the promulgation of life as a struggle— with death as our most implacable (and unconquerable) adversary. Despite our helplessness to avoid the inevitable passage into, as Hamlet says in his unforgettable soliloquy, that "undiscover'd country from whose bourne no traveller returns," we are nevertheless inclined to align ourselves with Dylan Thomas, who offered the following counsel in his memorable poem: "Do not go gentle into that good night... Rage, rage against the dying of the light."

It is a measure of the peculiar pathology of the Western mind at this juncture in its history that we are so resolutely terrified, not only of the ultimate transition to the world beyond, that ultimate step across the threshold into nonbeing, but also of that penultimate stage of existence, the autumn of our years. Our response to it, at least since the 1950s with the advent of a now-monolithic youth culture, has been to gradually reconfigure adulthood as protracted adolescence, to stave off even the appearance of maturity by any means—surgical, chemical, cosmetic, spiritual, dietary, physical—at our disposal. Society's upper echelons are replete with peculiarly immature, artificially youthful "adults" in their fifth and sixth decades of life who fail to embody a gravitas appropriate to their time of life and display little wisdom or moderation. Their aging can be observed to be anything but graceful.

This channel encodes our individual response to this inescapable fact of human mortality. If we have the capacity to envision our inevitable demise as an intrinsic aspect of existence, then we are more inclined to see ourselves as participating in a benign universe and capable of opening to unconditional love. All organic life-forms on this sphere partake of this perennial cycle of birth, increase, ripening, decline, and death; it is folly to pretend otherwise. One of the major responsibilities of the elder members of a group is to mentor the young and nourish them spiritually. One sees precious little of such mentoring from older generations at present.

It seems that the challenge embodied in this meridian is one of surrender. The ebbing away of our relentless Yang nature in later life affords us the opportunity to become more fully attuned with the Yin aspect of our being—to become still, serene, harmonious, and reflective. This surrender is not a defeat; it presents, rather, a potential release from the obsessive outward striving of our ever-more-imbalanced Yang civilization, through which we can extricate ourselves from the perennial "hamster's wheel" of the need to compete, to overcome, to surpass, to win at all costs. How exhausting this must be; if one were only sufficiently conscious to identify it and stop the suicidal juggernaut in its tracks.

As the paired channel to the Chong, Yin Wei Mai is also concerned with questions of identity. However, the Yin Wei focuses less on physical endowment and functioning associated with heredity, and rather more on individual motivations of soul development. It relates to the determination of one's life purpose and how one goes about ascertaining the meaning of life in a given incarnation.

While the Chong, with its archetypal idea of repeating patterns, relates to the dysfunction of obsessive/compulsive behaviors and addictions, Yin Wei speaks to a more profound desire to escape from the burdens of oppressive memories, both cellular and those engendered by their individual tribulations.

Yang Wei Mai

Yang Wei, in keeping with the outward expression of Yang, is more directly involved in the perception that as we age, in addition to the diminishment of our physical capacities, we experience a lessening of potentials available to us. Generally, with the enthusiasm and energy of youth, individuals in their teens and early twenties journey into larger society perceiving potentially unlimited possibilities. In this period of the apex of Yang vitality, setbacks are more readily viewed as merely temporary challenges. However, frustration with the nature of an initial career choice may cause a person to abandon that path; this may then raise the daunting specter of failure and the self-judgment that is its inevitable adjunct. How can they successfully overcome the challenges that will inevitably present themselves—continued survival and the maintenance of a sense of self-worth? Do they possess the courage to pursue their more authentic passion and strike out upon a new path, one more in alignment with the soul's purpose?

The master point of Yang Wei Mai is TH-5, and when considering the significance of the Triple Heater (TH), more profound metaphysical implications of this channel become apparent. The Triple Heater, or Triple Burner, is synonymous with the three Jiaos (San Jiao), alchemical furnaces that the ancient Chinese situated within the torso.

In both Eastern and Western alchemical practices, the fundamental operation aims for liberation of spiritual essence from its imprisonment in the dense matter of physical incarnation, either by physical or metaphorical means. The alchemist seizes upon the *prima materia*, the raw material of their experiments—the ignoble, base, unrefined stuff of ordinary existence, cast off, despised, ignored, usually black in hue, signifying its seemingly unredeemable nature—and casts it into a retort, a sealed furnace. Once therein, they subject it to intense heat, and the undistinguished lump of dreck gradually undergoes a series of transformations. The end result of this process is to burn off the dross and refine the anima, the spirit, of this *materia* into, ideally, the exalted state of gold, the metal of the Sun. The keyword here is transcendence, and we can certainly draw an analogy between the alchemical *opus* and the journey of life.

One of the challenges of a life lived as a spiritual pilgrimage lies in our continuing ability to reinvent ourselves, particularly as we reluctantly arrive at midlife, at which time the frailties of our physical nature become more readily apparent. Many individuals are disheartened by those first inklings of impending mortality, and it is here that we witness those stereotypical behaviors, the vain strivings after a lost youth, that are associated with midlife crises.

Often it becomes necessary to confront individual failures, although one should keep in mind that the definition of success agreed upon by societal consensus is unnecessarily narrow. Part of the emotional spectrum of authentic maturity includes the wisdom to recognize that all life experience is of value. The setbacks that we encounter in our vain pursuit of ambition frequently facilitate those course corrections necessary to align ourselves with higher purpose. Furthermore, not everything that is of enduring value in this world is guaranteed to make us wealthy or famous; there are other rewards to be accrued by remaining true to one's passion. Alchemical gold cannot be readily deposited in one's bank account.

Living a life informed by spiritual integrity and authenticity is, for the majority of those who eventually pursue it, never accomplished by means of a straightforward trajectory. The learned fear of failure, however irrational, may prevent us from having the courage to reinvent ourselves in midlife and risk a further immersion in those alchemical fires of transformation, from whence we may emerge yet again like the phoenix, reborn from the ashes of our former existence.

Chapter 4

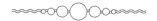

Anti-Exhaustion Treatments: Anchoring the Ying

All great changes are preceded by chaos.

Author unknown

In this chapter, we will address postnatal Qi (energy), as opposed to prenatal Qi, which relates to our genetic blueprint and the Eight Extraordinary meridians.

Postnatal Qi is to be distinguished from our inherited essence, as it bears little relation to our DNA; however, it does influence our genetic makeup. This energy finds its expression in the way we think, our dietary preferences and patterns, our exercise regimens, or lack thereof, our ability to relax, and the means that we choose to do so, our breathing patterns, and, in general, how we either maintain a state of balanced good health or undermine our well-being by self-destructive behavior and lifestyle choices.

Additionally, our experiences while growing up in our home of origin, and the relationships to family members, parents, and siblings, as well as our peers, have a noticeable impact upon this energy (Qi) and our capacity to interact with others beyond the family unit. It is important to question, take stock of, and be mindful of how we live, and love ourselves, in our daily interactions with the world.

A few questions may aid you in acquiring a better understanding of your postnatal Qi.

- Do you eat regular, nutritious meals, and nourish your Spleen (Earth element), or do you starve yourself so as to be thin, i.e., are you a victim of an eating disorder, either anorexia or bulimia?

⬥ Do you have a regular exercise regimen (Liver: Wood element), that is not abusive?

⬥ How do you relate to yourself and others? Do you have a significant other, or spouse/life partner (Heart: Fire element), or, if not, do you long for an authentic Heart connection?

⬥ Is your immune system strong (Lung: Metal element), or are you constantly succumbing to every mutated virus that comes along in your environment?

⬥ Most important, do you rest, sleep well, and revitalize the Kidney (Water element), which is the root/source of our longevity and continued health and well-being? Perhaps you are married to your smartphone or other electronic devices, or obsessed with social media so that you cannot rest or relax—ever.

These technology-addictive behaviors and the corresponding lack of proper rest can cause adrenal deficiency and exhaustion. Many of us these days are "running on empty," like a car without sufficient fuel, or an electric car lacking a proper charge. If you constantly feel that you are physically exhausted, emotionally taxed, with very little time to "be," you are like a hamster spinning an endless wheel. Or to cite an example closer to home, you're stuck on the treadmill at your "health" club, running without hope of relief from the monotonous effort of the task, never getting anywhere.

Life marches on in this case, but to the relentless and repetitive drumbeat of the crazy "zombie" who doesn't have the time to be vital, alive, creative, and joyous. Is that you?

If you answered yes to any of the above questions, the treatments proposed in this chapter will help you to target the root causes of psychospiritual and physical fatigue, from the inside out and the outside in, particularly relating to the deleterious impact of a toxic external environment with noise and air pollution, but also those conditions that may relate more to internal stressors.

We will explore in particular the dichotomy between a perception of the world via the eye vs. the ear, seeing vs. listening, and document to some extent the manner in which increasing dominance of the visual perspective, the *hypertrophy of the eye*, is creating a world that is ever more inimical to our continued survival as a species.

Special acupuncture points, the Yuan Source points, which are effective for addressing anxiety, anger, sadness, and depression, will be introduced. Post-traumatic stress syndrome (PTSS) is all too prevalent in our society at present. Transverse Yang Luo points will be coupled with the Yin Yuan Source points to deal with digestion, lifestyle issues, and psycho-emotional imbalances.

Considerations of sacred geometry will form the basis of an adjunct treatment with tuning forks and/or acupuncture needles, an approach that will further restore balance and alleviate the symptoms of the previously listed conditions.

Hang on to your hats—this chapter is full of information and practical recommendations for you and your patients.

Yuan Source Points

Each of the 12 primary channels has a Yuan Source point, where it is said the original Qi surfaces and lingers. In the *Classic of Difficulties*, we read the following:

> The dynamic Qi below the navel (Dantien) between the Kidneys [is the basis] of human life, and the root of the twelve channels is known as the original Qi. The Sanjiao is the envoy of original Qi... The term "source" is an honorary name for Sanjiao, therefore the places where it resides are known as the Yuan Source [points].[1]

Functions and Usage of the Yuan Source Points

- These points relate directly to the prenatal Qi.

- They can be evaluated by palpation because they reflect the prenatal Qi of each organ.

- They tonify Yin and Yang organs.

- The Yin Source points directly affect the organs. The *Spiritual Pivot* suggests that Source points can treat the imbalances of the organs directly.

- The Yang Source points dispel excess pathogens, such as wind, cold, etc.

Luo Connecting Points ————————————————

The Luo point of one meridian flows to the Yuan Source point of its complementary meridian. This relationship permits both meridians to balance each other, i.e., the practitioner can draw off excess Qi from one meridian and direct it to the other, to address a deficiency.

Functions and Usage of the Luo Connecting Channel

- Tonify the Luo point on the deficient meridians or sedate the Luo point on the excess meridians.

- Luo points normally tonify the Yin organs.

- In Yang organs, Luo points disperse or expel excess pathogenic factors.

- Luo meridians and their points do not treat pathology, rather they hold it in place.

- An imbalance in the body begins to incubate in the blood and fluids.

- The Twelve Regular meridians each have a specific point to access the Luo, which allows the patient to release what has been internalized, when they are ready to do so.

- Luo channels address Ying Qi, blood, and body fluids. Therefore, they can be used to address:

  - emotional issues

  - digestive imbalances

  - lifestyle issues.

- Luo channels communicate and connect with their Yin/Yang pairs and their companion meridians.

- Luo points hold the pathogen in check and prevent depletion of Ying Qi, blood, body fluids, and Jing.

Luo Meridian Imbalances

An external pathogenic influence (EPI) can invade the body by means of its fluids and/or blood. In clearing this heat from the patient's body, the pathogen can be released.

Anti-Exhaustion Yuan Source/Luo Treatment: Points and Indications

In the following constitutional treatments, Yin Yuan Source points are coupled with Yang Luo points. In the *Spiritual Pivot*, the Yin Yuan Source points are directly related to the organ systems, because original Qi arises from these points. This is the reason why Shudo Denmei-sensei, a noted expert in meridian therapy, always palpates and needles Source points when his diagnostics indicate that a particular organ is weak and needs support.

He also looks for changes in the skin: swelling, flaccid skin, redness, cysts and nodules, broken blood vessels, a bluish tinge, varicose veins, dips in the skin, i.e., a place where the skin is sunken—"kyo," or deficient, in Japanese treatments.

In review, the Yang Luo points hold pathogenic factors (illness) in check, using postnatal Qi—Ying Qi, blood, body fluids, and Jing. Synergizing the Yin Yuan Source points, which balance the Zang (Yin) organs, i.e., the Heart, Liver, etc., with the Yang Luo Connecting points, gives the patient time to process and release internalized emotions and digestive problems, and to explore alternative healthy lifestyle options.

The following Yin Yuan Source/Yang Luo treatment pairs and their relevant psycho-emotional imbalances are highlighted for treatments with the Acutonics Ohm® Unison tuning forks and/or acupuncture needling.

Wood Element
See Chapter 7 for the qualities of the Wood element.

- Yin Yuan Source point: Liv-3 Taichong, Great Rushing

- Yang Luo point: GB-37 Guangming, Bright Light

Liv-3 Taichong is located on the dorsum of the foot in the hollow distal to the junction of the first and second metatarsal bones. The source of Yuan Qi gathers at this point; you can use it to treat anger, anxiety, depression, headaches, premenstrual syndrome (PMS), bloating, cramps, and mood swings prior to menses. It clears thinking and releases frustration and/or jealousy. It also balances an overexcited, agitated person.

GB-37 Guangming is 5 cun directly above the tip of the lateral malleolus, on the anterior border of the fibula. This is the empirical point for treating the eyes and vision; it addresses and brightens both physical and psychospiritual sight. It also regulates the Liver, reduces heat in the Liver/Gall Bladder, and stimulates the anterior pituitary gland. It allows a person to be flexible, evokes a clear vision of the future, and aids in decision-making.

Fire Element
See Chapter 7 for qualities of the Fire element.

- Yin Yuan Source point: Ht-7 Shenmen, Spirit Gate

- Yang Luo point: SI-7 Zhizheng, Branch of the Upright

Ht-7 Shenmen is located on the radial side of the flexor carpi radialis muscle in the depression on the ulnar (pinky finger) side of the transverse crease of the wrist. Ht-7 is considered the home of the Spirit and is an essential point for treating all mental problems and deficiencies relating to the Heart. It calms the mind, eases stress and anxiety, aids with poor memory, and can be used to treat more serious issues, such as manic depression and dementia. Spirit Gate regulates the entry and exit into the Heart chamber. If this entrance is closed, Spirit is unavailable to calm a restless, anxious mind.

SI-7 Zhizheng is on the forearm, 5 cun above SI-5 Yanggu, Yang Valley, at the wrist. This Luo point on the Small Intestine meridian has a profound effect of regulating and calming spirit, and it is indicated for fear, fright, and extreme anxiety.

Earth Element
See Chapter 7 for qualities of the Earth element.

- Yin Yuan Source point: Sp-3 Taibai, Supreme White

- Yang Luo point: St-40 Fenglong, Abundant Bulge

Sp-3 Taibai is located on the medial side of the foot in the depression proximal and inferior to the head of the first metatarsal bone. This horary point represents Earth within Earth, and fosters a sense of groundedness, stability, connectedness, and richness within oneself. When imbalanced, damp issues arise, such as confused thinking, no appetite, congestion causing abdominal bloat, diarrhea, constipation, problems in the blood, Spleen deficiency, and prolapses of the uterus, bladder, etc. A person with a deficient Spleen may experience dissatisfaction and become melancholy and pensive.

St-40 Fenglong is found on the lower leg, 8 cun superior to the lateral malleolus (ankle bone), and 8 cun is roughly the halfway point between the ankle and the knee. This point encourages abundance, richness, joy, and satisfaction in life and work. Bountiful energy and nourishment are possible when connected to our bodies and Earth. You can lift a dissatisfied patient's spirit by using acu-sound treatments on St-40 Fenglong.

When a person is ungrounded and out of sync with their body, serious psychospiritual imbalances may develop, including seeing ghosts, insanity (Phlegm Misting the Mind), obsessions, nightmares, inappropriate laughter, and manic depression.

Metal Element
See Chapter 7 for qualities of the Metal element.

- ◼ Yin Yuan Source point: Lu-9 Taiyuan, Supreme Abyss

- ◼ Yang Luo point: LI-6 Pianli, Veering Passage

Lu-9 Taiyuan is located on the palmar side of the transverse crease of the wrist, in the small depression at the lateral side of the radial artery, which is on the thumb side of the hand. Use this point for a patient who is in a state of profound despair and depression. It is a revival point, a Hui meeting point of the vessels, which influences blood circulation and replaces instability with nourishment, security, and love.

When Qi is deficient and blood is not circulating in the body, it will stagnate in the Heart and chest, causing agitation, Heart pain, and in more serious manifestations, manic raving. Since blood unites the body and spirit, "stuck" blood can contribute to severe psycho-emotional problems.

LI-6 Pianli is 3 cun above LI-5 Yangxi, Yang Stream, on the line joining LI-5 Yangxi and LI-11 Quchi, Pool at the Crook. This point presents another way for the patient to release imbalances. The name, Veering

Passage, refers to the idea that this way is less traveled; it is a winding, veering path that has less in the way of obstructions. LI-6 is excellent for treating mental confusion, anxiety, fears, constant talking, insanity, and suicidal tendencies. It also helps to release heat, expels wind, regulates the water passage, and addresses nosebleeds, tinnitus, dim vision, and facial edema. In combination with its Yuan Source point, Lu-9 Taiyuan, the practitioner can address pathological symptoms of sadness.

Water Element
See Chapter 7 for qualities of the Water element.

- Yin Yuan Source point: Kid-3 Taixi, Supreme Stream

- Yang Luo point: Bl-58 FeiYang, Soaring Upwards

Kid-3 Taixi is located in the depression between the medial malleolus and the Achilles tendon. Here, Taixi becomes a stream and washes away the emotion of fear. It also tonifies Kidney Yang, regulates the uterus, supports the essence and the brain, strengthens the lower back and knees, treats insomnia and excessive dreaming, and reinforces the action of the Kidney grasping the Lung Qi.

Bl-58 FeiYang is on the lower leg, 7 cun directly above Bl-60 Kunlun, Kunlun Mountains, and about 1 cun inferior and lateral to Bl-57 Chengshan, Support the Mountain. This point brings order to scattered thoughts and feelings. It also releases fear that is deeply lodged in the cells of the body. It harmonizes body/mind/spirit and teaches the patient how to exert the appropriate amount of energy in accomplishing a task. It is a powerful point for cleansing mental/emotional imbalances. On a physical level, it expels wind from the TaiYang channel and alleviates pain along the channel; it helps with dizziness and treats rhinitis, chills and fever, sciatic pain, and brain disorders such as epilepsy.

What Is Sacred Geometry?

Our modern word *geometry* derives from an original Greek word that means "measurement of the Earth," which is conventionally known as surveying. The Greek mathematician Euclid (c. 325–265 BCE) was the first to summarize the theorems and axioms of plane, i.e., two-dimensional, geometry, in his book *Elements*. Geometry was considered sacred when it was believed to please the gods and goddesses; a temple was holy if it was constructed according to certain proportions and oriented in a specific direction.

The belief that numbers and proportions were imbued with qualitative, archetypal significance, rather than being merely quantitative, appears to have been more or less universal in the ancient world, but in the West, this philosophy originated with the legendary Pythagoras, the original philosopher. As was discussed in Chapter 1, numbers were of paramount importance to the Pythagoreans; indeed, they were nothing less than the fundamental constituents of the cosmos. Divinity was believed to be reflected in both the visually perceived symmetries of the heavens and the less tangible, mysterious attributes of musical tone. The association of proportion with the divine extended to the creation of sacred spaces that embodied archetypal principles; the Greek architects of these edifices employed their understanding of the nascent science of geometry to fashion structures that were noumenal, conceptual, mathematical, and natural.

This linking of Heaven with Earth through the agency of sacred space was common to all ancient peoples; each culture sought this connection through scrupulous application of acceptable harmonies of number and proportion. They strove, above all, to align their efforts with divine will, as expressed through the movements of planetary bodies, the perpetual cycle of the seasons, and, in Chinese medicine, the Five Elements.

While we are invoking principles of sacred geometry in these specialized treatments presented below, we are not creating geometric shapes upon our patients' bodies according to ancient traditions. The three components involved in these treatments—healing sound, acupuncture, and the body itself—can be regarded as replicating the triune realms of Heaven, Earth, and Humanity. The Acutonics Ohm® forks engender Earth energy, the electricity of the needles calls forth fire from Heaven, and both of these forms of vibrational Qi are directed toward the patient, the embodiment of Humanity. Additionally, the psychospiritual Source/Luo points relate to the Five Elements.

Sacred Geometry Treatments Using the Source/Luo Points
The "V" Vortex Treatment

1. Needle the acupuncture Source/Luo points.

2. Resonate the Acutonics Ohm® Unison tuning forks three times at the base of the needle, so as to form a V with the stems; first, treat the Yuan Source point, and then the Luo point.

This powerful treatment balances and rejuvenates both Yin Yuan Source and Yang Luo Five Element organs.

The tip of the V resonates with *terra firma*, and the two arms of the V reach upward to embrace the cosmos.

You can also use the V configuration upon the points without needling; the combination of Earth frequency (Ohm) and the harmonious perfection of the unison is both simultaneously grounding and transporting.

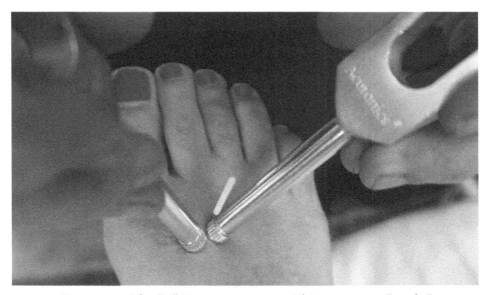

Figure 4.1 *The "V" Vortex treatment: This treatment "earths" the patient so that they can embody spiritual growth*

The Twister Treatment

1. Needle the Source/Luo points.

2. After striking the two Acutonics Ohm® Unison tuning forks, position them so that the vibrating tines, with their distinctive gold resonators, are angled toward the respective Source/Luo points and poised about 1 cun above the head of each needle.

3. Activate the needles by using a "twisting" technique, oscillating the forks back and forth, using your thumbs and index fingers. You can treat both Yuan Source and Luo points simultaneously.

The torqueing action of the Twister injects additional energy, further enlivening the sound waves that are activating the needle; metaphorically, you are "stirring the pot" by moving the Qi and stimulating the organs. This will also dispel blood stagnation, "stuck" blood, which can contribute to emotional imbalances.

The Three Treasures: Jing, Qi, and Shen

The human body is both electrical and vibrational; the resonant Qi of sound waves, which can be directed to every cell, connects us in a profound way to the Three Treasures—Jing, Qi, and Shen. Healing sound is holistic and integrative, and rekindles our cellular memory of undifferentiated wholeness. In its capacity to transform, it embraces both the practice of inner alchemy (Nei-dan), through its action at the deepest cellular level, and outer alchemy (Wai-dan), by harmonizing us with vibrations that have their ultimate source in planetary motion, the Music of the Spheres. The goal of Taoist alchemy is to nourish, enhance, and unify the Three Treasures.

Jing, Essence: Earth

Jing represents our prenatal, ancestral Qi. This genetic level rules bone, bone marrow, and Kidney essence. In China, a person with strong bone structure is considered to have powerful Jing and possesses great potential for good health, greater longevity, and the achievement of worldly success.

Qi, Energy: Humanity

This Qi aspect of the Three Treasures refers to postnatal Qi as it manifests in our lifestyle choices, i.e., what we eat, drink, think, feel, and hold sacred. Humanity is the bridge between Earth and Heaven, firmly grounded and yet aspiring to grasp the infinite. "We are all in the gutter, but some of us are looking at the stars."[2]

Shen, Spirit: Heaven

Shen represents spirit, the light that emanates from the eyes; it is an outward reflection of the compassionate heart. This Shen also links us to the crown chakra and the acupuncture point Du-20 Baihui, Hundred Meetings. As the medieval mystic Meister Eckhart wrote, this sacred place is "beyond the Godhead." Shen transports us into the present moment, permitting us to transcend preoccupations, grudges, blame, and our personal problems. It fosters a sense of timelessness, a quality of being totally present. This touches upon the Taoist philosophy of immortality, or, at least, greater longevity.

The Three Treasures Treatment

1. Needle the Source/Luo points.

2. Activate the Acutonics Ohm® Unison tuning fork combination.

   - Jing: resonate the forks at the base of the needle, three times.

   - Qi: resonate the middle of the needle, three times.

   - Shen: resonate about 1 cun above the needle, three times.

   - Make a note of when the vibration stops and at which of the three positions; return to that level, and resonate it an additional three times.

If the Jing level stops vibrating quickly, the patient may be ungrounded, or does not want to be in their body. Perhaps they were abused or sexually violated. This lack of grounding weakens the Qi and cuts off the connection to Heaven and the Shen.

If the Qi, middle area stops vibrating quickly, the patient's energy is low; they lack stamina and enough vitality to interact with the wider world. They may have poor dietary habits or suffer from eating disorders. Conversely, they could be addicted to food, drugs, or other substances.

As noted, the Shen level is about 1 cun above the needle; if the spirit is low, the patient may have experienced the loss of a loved one or be suffering from a serious illness themselves. Their Shen will appear to be dimmed, not vibrant or alive... You can readily observe this dullness in the eyes. These individuals are not present.

These Source/Luo sacred geometry treatments are very effective in addressing the root causes of our physical and psychospiritual fatigue manifesting in our inner emotional landscape.

Equally deleterious in their impacts are outer stressors, such as noise and air pollution, global warming, and environmental toxins, and electromagnetic frequency (EMF) wave sickness, due to microwave towers, the omnipresence of wireless communications networks, computers, etc. In this next section, we wish to focus further upon the impact of portable communications devices, particularly smartphones, which have come to assume a dominant focus in many people's lives, further skewing the nature of human interaction toward the visual, degrading the quality of our personal interactions, eroding our moral sensibilities, and rewiring our brains in the process.

Struggling to Be Heard in a Visually Dominated World —

The blind are more understanding than the deaf, because hearing exerts a direct influence on the formation of moral character, which is not immediately true of what is seen. The human soul can also become diffused by way of the eye whereas what is heard results in focus and concentration.

Aristotle

The Hypertrophy of the Eye

"Early, i.e., more primitive, humans...were primarily focused on hearing. Viewed 'historically,' the eye is the winner."[3] Our civilization has entered upon an era which is characterized by author Joachim-Ernst Berendt as being dominated by an "ocular hypertrophy."[4] In the past few decades, visual and other communications technology has all but transformed

Earth, and in ways that few of us could have imagined in the more tranquil days predating the arrival of the first black-and-white television sets. Those antediluvian apparatuses, for the first time, afforded the average person an electronic glimpse for a few hours a day of the wider world, beyond the previously circumscribed confines of family and community. Now, less than a century later, an increasing percentage of citizens in the industrialized nations are inhabitants of a global village or, given the increasingly minute virtual distances that separate us electronically, perhaps global *condominium* would be a more apt description. This phenomenon has been made largely possible by the institution of the Internet and further facilitated by the ready availability of convenient devices that provide instantaneous access to the same.

Many benefits have accrued to humankind in the wake of the Internet revolution and our entry as a species into the Information Age; however, we cannot overlook, as well, the potentially devastating impact of this increasingly one-sided emphasis upon the visual over the aural. For many of you, immersed in the mainstream, this distinction, and the implications thereof, will be somewhat mystifying. However, if you are to work effectively with healing sound, these differences are crucial, and you must begin to disentangle yourself from your unwitting immersion in this "brave new world" of the eye. It is important that you learn how to balance the senses.

A Study in Contraries

The eye and the ear present us with two contradictory views of reality, because they are diametrically opposed in their nature. The ancient Chinese saw the eye as being a Yang, male organ, and associated it with the Wood element. There are a number of excellent reasons for such a categorization. To begin with, it seems reasonable to construe the function of "seeing" as being an activity of engagement; our eyes are constantly scanning, gazing greedily at the world around us, gathering images for the optic nerve to transmit to the brain, which then synthesizes a simulacrum of reality from its binocular input that seems coherent. There is nothing contemplative or passive about this welter of outer-directed energy; one might argue that the eye seeks to conquer reality for the individual consciousness, to tame it, bring it to heel, so that the brain may assert its dominion over what it perceives.

In this manner, the eye separates us from the world; we peer outward at our surroundings from the twin apertures in our face, and the I, through the medium of the eye, becomes entirely cognizant of what is not-I. Thus, vision is a reductive and discriminatory faculty; in subjecting reality to our inveterate scrutiny, we also impose upon it our judgment, which may be anything but impartial.

In keeping with this idea of dominion, there is also a quality of ownership associated with the human perception of images; of course, this is entirely reflected in the commercial aspect of the art world. Visual artifacts, whether they be paintings or sculptures, depending on their provenance, are routinely auctioned for vast sums, so greatly exceeding what they would have commanded in the instant of their creation that it beggars belief.[5] This is because those enterprising capitalists with the requisite net worth can claim, given the appropriate outlay of funds, that they now possess these *objets d'art*. They can, if they choose, squirrel them away in secure vaults in the privacy of their opulent homes and reserve contemplation of their singular beauties for themselves, and perhaps their intimates, alone; given a later philanthropic bent, they might deign to endow a museum with their priceless possession.

This is not the case with compositions involving musical tones; no one can "own" a Beethoven symphony, a Puccini opera, an art song, a piano concerto, etc., even if they eventually acquire the autograph score of the same. These tonal creations only reside on the printed page *in potentia*; they are not fully realized until they are performed, and only endure within those comparatively brief instants of time during which the assembled musical forces—symphony orchestra, opera singer, instrumentalist—bring them into existence within an appropriate acoustic space; once these vibrations, no matter how transcendent, die away into the inevitable silence, they persist only as faint echoes within the soul of the listener. This evanescence remains an essential attribute even of music that has been recorded; after the recording stops, the only way to recapture the desired sounds is to reawaken them anew through the wonders of technology.

Moreover, reproduction of music by electronic means does not replicate the actual experience of live performance. To translate the tonal input into a somewhat durable (and increasingly portable) format, one that can be activated at will so as to recreate the desired sounds, the original vibrations must be compressed to accommodate the narrow confines of the recording medium; with each subsequent technological innovation, the compression of the auditory signal in the interest of easier storage and transfer removes some of the essential acoustic quality.

Rudolf Steiner, the anthroposophist and mystic, wrote that live music was vivified by the presence of nature spirits or elementals; in the days of the long-playing record, he said that one could observe the elementals crushed beyond recognition in the grooves of its surface. One can only hazard a guess as to what the elementals' condition might be as a consequence of a transfer of music from analog to digital media. Thus, when we listen to recorded music, with our iPods, on our smartphones, with iTunes, etc., our ears are subjected to a performance in which the transcendent spiritual essence of the music in question is no longer extant.

"*Armonia aphanes phaneros kreisson.*" (Hidden harmony is mightier than what is revealed.)[6] It is perhaps for this reason, as the Greek philosopher Heraclitus suggests, that many ancient cultures, not being able to capture sound to be experienced again at a future date, regarded listening as the *summa* of man's sensory faculties, in that the ephemeral quality of auditory stimuli hinted at realities beyond the physical realm. The ancient practitioners of these emergent sound technologies sought to establish balance, personal and communal, through an immersion in transcendent frequencies. As did the ancient Chinese—they believed that the judicious use of sound would, by its very nature, engender a harmony that encompassed the entirety of the community, the kingdom, the empire. These agencies were utilized to establish a continuum of vibration between the supernal frequencies of the heavens, the abode of divinity, and the quotidian realm of human beings. Pythagoras referred to these cosmic tones as the Music of the Spheres, and similar notions regarding the harmonious connection between macrocosm and microcosm were posited by the ancient Chinese.

Plato, who in the centuries after the emergence of the Pythagorean doctrine of celestial harmony became its principal advocate, particularly in his dialogue *Timaeus*, which describes the creation of the universe in purely musical terms, also saw the reestablishment of this vital connection between human beings, living in a fallen state here on Earth, and the heavens, as essential:

> The world soul is created with perfect harmonies inherent in its structure, but when this becomes embodied in human beings, the process of infusion results in distortion and upheaval and therefore the

human soul needs to be "reminded" of the perfect harmonies it once enjoyed. It can then realign itself with the cosmos, and ultimately with the divine mind itself.[7]

The ear, through its capacity to perceive these otherworldly tones, provides us with a direct conduit to the essence of divinity. This is consistent with its Yin nature, as posited by the ancient Chinese and others. The ear is a receptacle, analogous to the female sex organ in its configurations; in ancient cultures, it was often likened to a seashell. The eye, by comparison, which thrusts out into the world, has been depicted as an arrow, demonstrating clearly its phallic nature.[8]

The ear was associated by the Chinese with the Water element, and it has an intrinsic linkage in its configurations with the Kidney organ. Sound must travel *to* the ear, which waits patiently, passively, for the arrival of the desired vibrations. In contrast with the eye, which establishes a polarity, a duality, between the observer and the observed, the ear's absorption and processing of sound waves is essentially an integral function; the perception of tone does not occur at a remove, and the physiological responses of the listener are entrained with the origin of the sound. Thus, the individual reaction to auditory impulses facilitates an energetic rapport between the resonator and the listener.

This cannot be said of that which is seen; there is always a subjective feeling of distance that accompanies our viewing of something in our immediate environment, no matter how minute that separation might be. Conversely, while we may perceive that a sound is closer or farther away, due to its amplitude in a given moment, our ears are capable of identifying the source of this stimulus without actively seeking it.

Consistent with the Yang nature of the eye, its essential function as a receptor of light can be construed as providing fuel for the relentless mechanism that now drives our hypervisual, overly technologized society, the Internet. The speed of light, 186,000 miles per second, is the fastest velocity in the known universe, and it is certainly arguable that the latest innovation in the transmission of data over the Internet, fiber*optic* networks, further facilitates the quasi-instantaneous transfer of visual images. Our civilization is speeding up, and we have increasingly little tolerance for forms of communication that are not in accord with that relentless pace. Although it's becoming more difficult for us to maintain our equilibrium in the face of this overwhelming surfeit of electronic signals, many people are hopelessly addicted to the "buzz" that they receive when they interact with these new technologies.

Unlike the waves and particles of light, sound vibrations are remarkably slow: only 1126 feet per second in air. The difference between the velocity of the two types of signal is on the order of magnitude of 850,000:1. By comparison with seeing, hearing is a leisurely activity, one that predisposes an individual to take time. Moreover, listening is a capacity of our human senses that requires a relative degree of stillness, otherwise, we may lose contact with the source of the sound. We can be hurtling past a landscape in an automobile at speeds ranging from 60 to 100 mph, but, although the shifting topography may scroll past our gaze, at no point is the transmission of the visual input interrupted. How quickly, in contrast, does that elusive FM channel on our antiquated car radio disappear out of range—unless the station has an incredibly powerful transmitter—without the benefit of geosynchronous satellites?

> *The eye says I.*
>
> Krishnamurti

There seems to be an intrinsic linkage in the human psyche between the eyes and the sense of ego consciousness; it is certainly true that, symbolically, consciousness may be characterized as the emergence of light from the primordial darkness, and it is the eyes of human beings that have the capacity to perceive this light. This miracle of our evolutionary process as a species is reflected in many creation myths. However, this embrace of light at the expense of darkness also sunders us from our instinctual way of being; we lose our capacity to be cradled in the bosom of nature and leave the earth behind to dwell in sterile constructs of our own fashioning.

The parallel between vision and the ego is also embedded in our vocabularies; Table 4.1 provides a few samples from European languages of the remarkable similarities between the two words.

Table 4.1 The organ of vision and ego consciousness

Language	The organ of vision	Individual (ego) consciousness
English	Eye	I
French	Oeil	J'ai
Italian	Occhio	Io
German	Auge	Ich

Visual Technology and Its Impact on Empathy and Authentic Communication

> Human beings, with their disproportionate emphasis on seeing, have brought on the excess of analysis, of rationality and abstraction, whose breakdown we are now witnessing. In the age of television [and by extension, all visual technology] seeing people have allowed themselves to be led *ad absurdum*. ... Living almost exclusively through the eyes has led us to almost not living at all.[9]

As ear people, we have witnessed, with some distress, the increasing dominance of visually centered technology upon the waking lives of virtually everyone in the Western world. American adults spend more than 11 hours per day watching, reading, listening to or simply interacting with media, according to a new study by market-research group Nielsen.[10] The far-reaching impact of this constant and, invariably, insatiable interfacing with iPads, iPhones, computer screens of all kinds, televisions, etc., is only just now being assessed by scientists and social psychologists, but the implications are more than a bit disturbing.

In his meticulously researched and provocative book *The Shallows*, Nicholas Carr[11] has reported that even a minimal exposure to the Internet begins to rewire the brain, activating a hitherto largely dormant area, the dorsolateral prefrontal cortex. This is an area that seems to thrive on primate-based distraction, what we might appropriately label the "monkey mind." It is likely that this particular locus of the brain has been largely silent for the entirety of our evolution as a species, and that, with its eruption into life, and the subsequent addiction to the atomization of information that feeds it, many of us are losing our capacity for the type of deep contemplation that has been the fountainhead for many of our most inspired and creative innovators and thinkers. With this increasing deficit of the individual capacity for sustained rational thought, there is an ancillary loss of empathy and affect that is a concomitant of the fractured and non-intimate communication that is a hallmark of these new technologies. Who would have imagined that the telephone, that revolutionary artifact of the early 20th century, one that permitted people to converse at vast distances, approximately a century later would increasingly be used to send nonverbal, fragmentary bits of degenerated text?

Mr. Carr, an inveterate and enthusiastic adopter of all the latest gadgets and apps, a blogger, etc., the quintessential "wired-in" champion and observer of much of what Silicon Valley has to offer, found that he had to disconnect entirely from these sources of distraction, with their incessant demands upon his attention, because his addiction to being connected made it impossible for him to focus on the solitary, concentrated task of writing a book: "The very way my brain worked seemed to be changing. ... I began worrying about my inability to pay attention to one thing for more than a couple minutes. ... I missed my old brain."[12]

We can personally attest to the shortened attention spans, inability to retain information, etc., that are entirely characteristic of many of the current generation of students; these effects are not necessarily confined to millennials: "In a talk at a recent Phi Beta Kappa meeting, Duke University professor Katherine Hayles confessed, 'I can't get my students to read whole books anymore.' Hayles teaches *English*; the students she's talking about are students of *literature*."[13]

A dear friend of ours has opined that, were she to lose her smartphone, it would be the equivalent of a lobotomy; she has outsourced her memory to a device and would be cast adrift, without any moorings for her day-to-day activity. While both of us own smartphones as devices of contingency communication, we do not participate in smartphone culture or social media, except to promote our various business endeavors.

While it is beyond the purview of this book to dwell at length on this subject, we wish to point out that it is the Yang nature of the eye, as the hyperactive conduit for this information to the brain, that facilitates this immersion in the superficiality and meaninglessness of much of the omnipresent visual culture. Many people confine their reading to skating along the surface of the Internet and are entirely content with the novelty and constraints of compressing argument and discourse into 280-character outbursts via Twitter or texting instead of engaging in direct face-to-face dialogue with their friends and intimate acquaintances—even if they are in close proximity to these individuals.

In our experience, the use of healing sound is a necessary palliative for those individuals who have become *ensnared* by the World Wide Web and its adjuncts. The choice of verb is quite deliberate; as Mr. Carr and others have described it, there is a decidedly insidious quality to the way that this technology, which has insinuated its fiberoptic tendrils into the intimate fabric of our lives, is ruthlessly splintering our consciousness. Sound therapy presents an opportunity for these fragmented souls to be still and receptive, to shut out the myriad distractions and demands for attention that enter in by way of the eye, letting their entire body resonate with frequencies that permit them to reharmonize the dissonance that permeates their lives.

The Acutonics Ohm® Unison tuning forks introduced in this book are noticeably effective in reconnecting people with Earth energy, reinforcing the Yin aspect of their lives, especially if they live in large cities, without contact with nature. The motive force of our global technocracy is primarily an electrical one that profoundly ungrounds us at every juncture, making us susceptible to a range of deleterious influences. The individual who is rooted in their own physical being, vital in their Qi, with the capacity to listen with discrimination to the promptings of their own inner wisdom, tuning out the cacophony of the Zeitgeist, is more likely to live a harmonious life—one in which there is an appropriate balance between receptivity and activity, rest and movement, compassion and discernment—maintaining the serenity of the Yin within the frenzy of the Yang that is the largely unavoidable essence of contemporary life.

Table 4.2 The qualities and functions of the eye vs. the ear

The eye	The ear
The eye compares and estimates.	The ear measures.
The eye seeks.	The ear finds.
The eye approximates and does not have an absolute visual sense.	The ear has the capacity for absolute hearing (perfect pitch).
The eye has one third as many connections to the brain.	The ear has three times as many connections to the brain.
Alpha rhythms[14] are not stimulated by the eye.	Sound waves can stimulate alpha rhythms.
The eye is Yang, male, aggressive, judgmental, and patriarchal.	The ear is Yin, feminine, receptive, sensual, and maternal.
The eye can perceive only one octave of light.	The hearing capacity of most human beings is ten octaves.
The eye scans repeatedly and makes errors (optical illusions).	The ear has but one opportunity to identify a sound; therefore, listening puts one more in the present moment and makes one less prone to errors.

Chapter 5

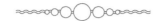

Harmonizing the Wei

Stay close to anything that makes you feel glad to be alive.

Hafiz

In Chapter 3, we introduced the Eight Extraordinary meridians, which relate to the Jing level of constitutional body treatments. These meridians are repositories for Jing, the clearest distillate of essence, fundamentally linked to the core of our individual identity. We provided some entirely new psychospiritual information concerning their function and introduced several treatments utilizing aspects of sacred geometry, as well as some practical insights as to the best use of our two treatment modalities, tuning forks and needles, when treating the Eight Extraordinary channels.

In presenting material on anti-exhaustion treatments in Chapter 4, our intention was to show various means for anchoring the Yin, using the Twelve Regular meridians, Source/Luo points, treatment of postnatal Qi, and incorporation by the patient of beneficial lifestyle changes.

In this chapter, our focus is on harmonizing the Wei Qi. We will introduce techniques for releasing the exterior, using the tendinomuscular meridians (TMM), which travel in the depressions and planes between the muscles and tendons. They are considered conduits of Wei Qi, because they protect the body from damp, wind, heat, cold, and trauma. They are located on the superficial aspect of the body and have the following characteristics.

- They overlap each other and involve more than one meridian.

- They are nourished by the Twelve Regular meridians.

⬥ They are responsible for the circulation of Qi and blood in the exterior of the body.

⬥ They can be used to treat imbalances of the muscles, joints, ligaments, and tendons.

⬥ Their symptomatology includes sprains, spasms, stiffness, restricted movement of the joints, muscle weakness due to overuse or injuries, or muscle tension caused by stress or trauma.

Trigger, motor, and "ashi" (tight, tender) points are identified through palpation of the muscles involved in the pattern.

What Are Trigger Points?

Myofascial trigger points are located in tissue that is compressed and tender. This gives rise to what is called a referred pain pattern, and they are customarily activated when a muscle remains in a shortened position for a long period of time or has been subjected to repetitive strain.

The late Janet G. Travell, M.D., recommended the use of a "snapping palpation" or rolling of the trigger point (muscle and/or fascia) between the fingertips to ascertain where it is most tender. When these points are needled, there is a jump, or fasciculation, which refers back to the attachment at the end of the muscle or muscle groups. Using a pecking needling technique stimulates and irritates the trigger point, and the shortened muscle usually jumps when the accumulated tension is released.

What Are Motor Points?

A motor point is a specific location where nerves enter into muscles (a neuromuscular junction). When these sites are needled, the muscle fires and resets its spindles, accompanied by a grabbing/gripping action. Information concerning this stimulation of the muscle spindle is transmitted to the central nervous system (CNS), which then instructs the muscle either to relax (if tight and contracted) or tighten (if flaccid or weak). The patient may feel a subjective sensation that is similar to "da Qi"—an achy feeling, a sensation of heat, or a grabbing of the needle. However, this response has been caused by the stimulation of the neuromuscular junction and should not be confused with the arrival of Qi.

Motor Points vs. Trigger Points

A motor point is usually treated when a muscle has become atrophied or when it is very tight. As it is a neuromuscular junction, it is needled via an acupuncture point (or points), however, it should be noted that it is an anatomical area characterized by the enervation of muscle. Each area can be in a slightly different place and will not be the same on both sides of the body (or face). It is imperative that the practitioner searches for the motor point and likewise recognizes that an individual patient's reaction to the stimulation of motor points may differ from side to side, depending upon the condition of the muscles. It should also be noted that some patients have slower CNS reactions to the needling of motor points, and the associated responses—achy feeling, release of heat, etc.—may take longer to register. Be patient with them and make sure that they experience the appropriate sensations as a result of the needling.

Some practitioners suggest that motor points and trigger points are identical. A trigger point can be located at the site of a motor point and may appear to be the same, but I have not found this to be the case. A trigger point is not usually situated in a neuromuscular junction, and they are located more superficially than motor points when palpated.

What Are "Ashi" Points?

The Japanese term *ashi* refers to a point that is tight and tender; these points may be either trigger points or motor points.

When performing Chinese medicine treatments as a licensed acupuncture professional and integrating motor and trigger points into your treatments, you are using acupuncture needles on the points and meridians of the body. Acupuncture is very effective for treating tendinomuscular issues, and many acupuncturists establish lucrative practices in the field of sports medicine.

I integrate tendinomuscular treatments in my practice on a regular basis and use these points for constitutional treatments, as well as more significant issues such as windstroke, Bell's palsy, postoperative neuropathies, and also temporomandibular joint dysfunction (TMJ). They are also effective in the treatment of a tight shoulder, sprained ankle, etc.

The Acutonics Ohm® Unison tuning forks can also be used in the treatment of TMJ and other constitutional syndromes, on both face and body points. Sensitive patients are extremely receptive to the application of the tuning forks, finding the approach soothing, nonthreatening, and effective.

Combining the two modalities is likewise a dynamic way to address these various issues. First use the tuning forks on the TMJ or other treatment points and then needle the patient afterwards. The treatment points will positively balance, open, and release quicker than if you simply used one or the other modality by itself. This will also make the experience more comfortable for the patient.

Please note: Do not insert acupuncture needles if you are not a licensed acupuncturist, trained in an accredited school for three-plus years.

Temporomandibular Joint Dysfunction (TMJ)

One of the most debilitating and painful of all facial syndromes is TMJ. TMJ manifests as an acute or chronic inflammation of the mastication (chewing) muscles. This pain can be accompanied by restricted jaw movement, clicking or popping of the joints, and myofascial pain. The muscles involved in this syndrome are the masseter, temporalis, and the medial and lateral pterygoids.

The temporomandibular joint itself relates to two muscles:

* the medial (internal) pterygoid muscle, which protracts and elevates the lower jaw and assists in the rotary motion while chewing

* the lateral (external) pterygoid muscle, which protrudes the mandible, pulls the articular disc forward, and likewise assists with the rotary motion of chewing.

These two joints both rotate and slide, which can contribute to wear and tear of bone and cartilage.

TMJ impacts the muscles, nerves, tendons, ligaments, bones, connective tissue, and teeth. Pain originates in the soft myofascial tissue, and TMJ can cause tinnitus, facial pain, and otalgia (pain in the ear).

Muscles

Clicking and popping of the joints can be caused by:

- overuse of the mastication (chewing) muscles

- chewing gum

- biting the fingernails, as well as pencils, pens, etc.

- cracking ice with one's teeth and then chewing it

- bruxism, i.e., clenching the jaw

- trauma or an accident, resulting from whiplash

- habitually holding the mandible too tight

- over-opening the jaw, as occurs, for example, in a dental treatment

- unusual speech patterns and chewing habits, for example, thrusting the jaw forward

- eating huge portions of food and overextending the opening of the jaw

- myofascial pain syndrome (trigger and motor points).

According to Dr. Travell, the masseter muscle can cause "unilateral tinnitus [ringing in the ears], which may arise from TMJ…and could be explained by the fascial connection between the TMJ and the middle ear." [1]

Teeth

Dysfunctions relating to the teeth can contribute to TMJ, such as:

- an impaired mobility due to bone and tooth loss

- overbite/underbite relating to chewing problems and disequilibrium of the jaw when chewing

- trismus; limitation of jaw movement

- myofascial pain and occultation of the teeth

- occlusal imbalances with the teeth.

Suggested Treatments and Personal Care

The following are some recommended strategies for the correction of dental imbalances resulting from facial trauma, accidents, and stress.

- Eliminate negative oral habits; use a mouth guard to prevent bruxism.

- Gentle stretching exercises for the jaw.

- Acupuncture/tuning fork treatments using myofascial trigger points and motor points.

- Cranio-sacral work in the mouth, targeting the masseter and pterygoid muscles.

- Stress reduction.

- Biofeedback.

- Physiotherapy.

- Psychotherapy: consult a therapist to help with the resolution of psycho-emotional issues such as anger, depression, or anxiety:

  - stress and anxiety can cause nocturnal bruxism, sustained muscular spasms, and contractions in the face and jaw.

- Chiropractic treatments.

- Low-level lasers may help with the pain of TMJ.

- Ultrasound treatments will contribute to increased blood flow and faster healing of affected tissues.

- Massage therapy.

- Microcurrent transcutaneous electrical nerve stimulation (TENS) treatments can help override the pain (see an acupuncturist or another healthcare professional).

Other Considerations

Genetic factors may contribute to the development of TMJ and other chronic pain syndromes. The coding for certain genes may be associated with a higher sensitivity to pain.

There is also evidence to suggest that estrogen levels may be a significant factor in the higher occurrence of TMJ in women. This is related to hormone fluctuations during ovulation or just prior to menstruation. Women who are postmenopausal may also develop TMJ if they are undergoing hormone replacement therapy (HRT).

The incidence of TMJ in women is approximately double that of men, and they are also more willing to seek treatments. Despite this, their symptoms are not easily resolved. The answer to this may lie in the fact that women are more sensitive to psycho-emotional stressors than men, as well as other genetic factors, including the variance in their estrogen levels.

However, it is likewise documented that six months prior to the onset of the first symptoms of TMJ, 50–70 percent of *both* women and men had experienced unanticipated and stressful events relating to their work, their personal finances, or their health, including the loss of a loved one or the failure of a relationship.

The first muscle associated with TMJ that we are going to introduce is the masseter. We recommend needling the motor points, neuromuscular junctions, to treat imbalances in this muscle.

Temporalis Muscle TMJ Treatment

While we recommend choosing one of the TMJ muscle treatments, depending upon your patient's signs and symptoms, *the temporalis muscle is always treated first.*

Table 5.1 The temporalis muscle

Functions	The temporalis muscle elevates the jaw, retracts the mandible, and clenches the teeth.
Nerve	The deep temporal branches of the anterior trunk of the mandibular division of the trigeminal nerve.
Treatment points	• GB-9 Tianchong, Heavenly Rushing, is above the ear in the depression 0.5 cun posterior to GB-8 Shuaigu, Leading Valley. Shuaigu is 1 cun above the apex or tip of the ear. • GB-10 Fubai, Floating White, is 1 cun from GB-9 Tianchong (see Figure 5.1). All of these points are located on the scalp and above the ear on the Gall Bladder meridian.

cont.

Needling techniques	Use a thicker needle for the scalp—a Seirin #3 (0.20, gauge 30 mm) is recommended. Palpate and locate GB-8 Shuaigu first, then palpate GB-9 Tianchong, which is 0.5 cun behind GB-8 Shuaigu. Then find GB-10 Fubai 1 cun from GB-9 Tianchong. Insert the needle obliquely, then angle it toward GB-9 Tianchong, and then thread it (connect it) to GB-10 Fubai. Treat the temporalis muscle bilaterally to prevent imbalances in the TMJ muscles, tension headaches, and migraines.
Tuning forks technique	Vibrate the Acutonics Ohm® Unison tuning fork combination on GB-9 Tianchong; then, after three seconds, move one of the forks to GB-10 Fubai, while the other fork remains in position. Treat three times on both sides of the scalp.

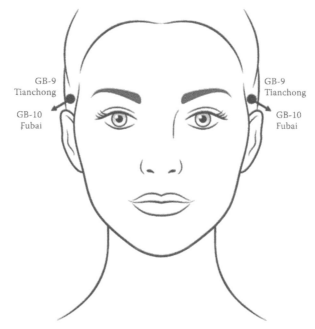

Figure 5.1 *The temporalis muscle: tightness in the temporalis muscle can cause tension headaches and/or migraines*

Masseter Muscle TMJ Treatment

Treating the masseter muscle helps to address:

⬧ bruxism (grinding the teeth)

⬧ chronic overwork

⬧ acute overload of the masseter muscle

- accumulated imbalances

- stress, anger, frustration, anxiety, and negative habits.

Table 5.2 The masseter muscle

Functions	Elevates the jaw; clenches the teeth.
Nerve	Masseteric nerve, from the anterior trunk of the mandibular division of the trigeminal nerve.
Treatment points	• Qianzheng, an extra point, is located 1 cun lateral from the middle of the earlobe. • St-6 Jiache, Jaw Bone, is located one fingerbreadth anterior and superior to the angle of the jaw, at the prominence of the masseter muscle. However, we are not needling this point directly, but using one acupuncture needle to stimulate the motor points on the jaw. Both points affect the fibers of the masseter muscle.
Needling technique	**Motor point #1: Qianzheng** Needle Qianzheng perpendicularly 0.5 cun; when you have your depth, angle the needle horizontally toward the center of the face. Pull back on the needle to see if the muscle grabs it. The patient may experience a subjective achy feeling or sensation of heat. Please be aware that the needle will not move from the insertion point and will not physically travel across the cheek toward the nose. It is important to elicit the grabbing response from the muscle when needling the motor point. You will also observe that if you attempt to retract the needle, the skin will pucker at the site of the insertion. **Motor point #2: St-6 Jiache** Pull back the needle and retract it without removing it from the patient's face, and then angle it straight down toward the masseter muscle. This motion should activate this second motor point, and the needle will not move beyond the site of the original insertion.
Tuning fork techniques	The tuning forks add a vibrational component to these TMJ treatments and are wonderful for needle-phobic patients. The treatment points are the same, but the approach is different. **Motor point #1: Qianzheng** Place both of the Acutonics Ohm® Unison tuning forks on the extra point Qianzheng and resonate them three times on this point. Then leave one of the pair on Qianzheng and move the other 1 cun toward the center of the face (follow the arrows in Figure 5.2). Execute the motion three times on each side of the face. **Motor point #2: St-6 Jiache** Resonate both forks on extra point Qianzheng once. Leave one fork on Qianzheng and move the other fork toward the center of the face 1 cun, as you did previously. Then, while the tuning forks are still vibrating, angle the second fork downward toward St-6 Jiache 1 cun (see Figure 5.2). Repeat this procedure three times on each side of the face.

If you are integrating both tuning forks and acupuncture needles, apply the forks first, three times, then needle the acupuncture points.

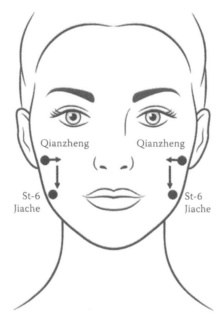

Figure 5.2 *The masseter muscle: TMJ imbalances manifest as tightness and pain in one or both of the muscles of the jaw*

Lateral and Medial Pterygoid Muscles TMJ Treatment

The paired pterygoids are the principal chewing muscles. Both assist with the rotary motion involved in chewing. Imbalances and tension in the pterygoids can give rise to a click in the jaw, which occurs when the mouth is opened. It is important for the cartilage in the TMJ joint to articulate and move backwards and forwards easily. A big click in the jaw indicates that the muscle is contracted, and the condyloid disc has slipped off the cartilage of the bone.

Table 5.3 The lateral and medial pterygoid muscles

Functions	The lateral (external) pterygoid protrudes the mandible and pulls the articular disc forward. The medial (internal) pterygoid protracts and elevates the lower jaw.
Nerves	The lateral pterygoid nerve is a branch of the anterior division of the mandibular nerve. The medial pterygoid nerve is from the mandibular division of the trigeminal nerve.
Treatment points	• St-7 Xiaguan, Below the Joint, is located at the lower branch of the zygomatic arch, in the depression anterior to the condyloid process of the mandible. • St-6 Jiache, Jaw Bone, is located one fingerbreadth anterior and superior to the angle of the jaw, at the prominence of the masseter muscle.
Needling techniques	The techniques involved with these muscles are similar to those for treating the masseter, except that you needle St-7 Xiaguan perpendicularly 0.5 cun; when you reach your depth, angle the needle transversely toward the center of the face. You will not reach the center of the face, but will remain in the same location where you inserted the needle. Make sure that the muscle grabs the needle. Then angle the needle downward toward St-6 Jiache, in the same way as you did for the masseter muscle.

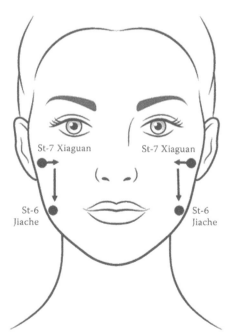

Figure 5.3 *The lateral and medial pterygoid muscles: imbalances of the pterygoid muscles are usually the underlying cause of a click on one side, or both sides, of the jaw*

Palpation and Discernment

It is important to decide which TMJ muscle needs treatment; always treat the temporalis muscle bilaterally first.

Masseter muscle:

⬦ Palpate the masseter muscle cross-fiber to discern if it is tight and which side is the tighter of the two. Needle and/or fork the side that is not as tight first. This will open up the tight side of the jaw and make the treatment more comfortable for the patient.

Pterygoid muscles:

⬦ Place the fingers of both hands on St-7 Xiaguan bilaterally and have the patient open their jaw to determine whether clicking noises occur on either or both sides. If so, this indicates that the pterygoid muscles must be treated, and that the TMJ is more severe, affecting the condyloid process of the jaw. In this case, needle and/or fork the side that is tight first, not the weak or clicking side. This releases tension and the pull on the weak side of the jaw.

Treat the temporalis muscle, then the pterygoids. If there is no click in the jaw, but just a tight or tender masseter muscle, start once again with the temporalis and then perform the needling protocol or resonate with the Acutonics Ohm® Unison tuning forks bilaterally on the masseter.

Bilaterally is the operative word! Do not just treat the affected side, but rather both sides, or your patient may experience discomfort. As human beings, our anatomical structure is essentially bilaterally symmetrical, but in the facial landscape, these paired muscles should never be treated in isolation. You should treat them as a single unit.

Conclusion

I have introduced material concerning trigger point needling in this chapter, but have chosen to highlight motor point treatments instead, because they are very effective, less invasive, and more comfortable for the patient. Motor point needling is also easier to explain in a written text. I recommend that you study with a master acupuncturist in a live seminar, not a webinar, to learn how to practice these valuable techniques. Nothing can take the place of authentic mentorship from a master teacher.

Earlier in the chapter, we discussed the differences between the two approaches, and the advantages of using both approaches. I utilize trigger points and motor points in my practice on a regular basis and achieve very good results.

In treating TMJ, it is important to ensure that the patient's neck and shoulders are free of tension, as well as the scalp (temporalis muscle). You should likewise be aware of the individual patient's stressors and emotional triggers.

Prior to working with the patient's TMJ, start with the Corpus Callosum Balancing treatment from Chapter 8, and thoroughly ground the patient with the Acutonics Ohm® Unison tuning fork combination. Utilize the Eight Extraordinary meridians to address the Jing, DNA level (see Chapter 3).

Remember that patients can have a hereditary predisposition to experience TMJ. I recommend opening the Belt meridian to address Gall Bladder/Liver imbalances, which can manifest as anger or frustration. Then, needle or fork the indicated points for TMJ imbalances. Later, you can add on other treatment protocols.

Chapter 6

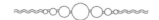

Facial Acu-Sound Protocols

It's never too late to be what you might have been.

George Eliot

In previous chapters, we have covered material relating to the three levels of constitutional treatment, providing you with an effective means to address those vital components of Jing (Eight Extraordinary meridians), Ying (Twelve Regular meridians; Source/Luo points), and Wei (TMJ treatments). In this chapter, we have laid the necessary groundwork to facilitate your engagement with the face from an aesthetic perspective, but we hasten to remind you that the face is not separate from the body. An authentic transformation, both of the facial landscape and of your patient on a psychospiritual level, is more readily achieved with a constitutional approach.

Perhaps you were waiting for just this moment…when you will learn two protocols designed to lift, tone, and balance the face and neck using the Acutonics Ohm® Unison tuning forks and/or acupuncture needles.

The first treatment is a balancing facial using just the Acutonics Ohm® Unison tuning fork combination. This protocol is purely vibrational, and you will learn specialized techniques for using these tuning forks on the face. As has been previously noted, the combination of the harmonious nature of the unison interval with the grounding energy of the Ohm Earth tone produces a synergetic effect that is relaxing and peaceful.

The second protocol targets "turkey wattles," the two cords that hang down from the front of the neck. These folds are reminiscent of Thanksgiving and, if you live in North America, our favorite American holiday bird, but those who develop them are not always thankful!

We will address these "wattles" with both tuning forks and motor point needling to ameliorate the appearance of a saggy, drooping neck. The muscle that is involved in the formation of these folds of skin is the platysma.

Some of you may have objections to what might be described as beauty treatments and perhaps, like many, you regard any such attention paid to one's appearance as vain and superficial. However, it seems indisputable that in our highly technologized and visual era, the face has become the equivalent of an organic calling card. Leaving aside purely aesthetic considerations, an increasing number of us are choosing to communicate with others by means of devices (and not just limited to smartphones) that have visual screens.

In our online webinar, *The Depression Suppression*, available on YouTube, we introduced the idea that such communication leads to the unconscious cultivation of what can be described as a false intimacy. In other words, when two people are engaging in a video chat on their smartphones, their faces, electronically rendered, are displayed in an apparent proximity on the screen that would not be considered appropriate in a nonvirtual interaction, unless they were a couple...or, at the very least, close friends. The impersonal and emotionless violation of personal space that is achieved in these tele-dialogues subjects the participants to a level of scrutiny that is extreme, leaving them open to potential negative judgment by others, as well as their own self-judgment, as many people are not at all pleased about how they look in these interactions.

By way of contrast, people in the entertainment world—movie and television actors, newscasters, emaciated models, etc., who loom large in our lives due to their presence on these screens—have every aspect of their appearance curated. They work out every day, spend hours in the makeup chair, and are arrayed in wardrobes carefully chosen to highlight their physical attractiveness, with hair meticulously arranged so that every follicle is firmly in place. Their livelihood is rooted in this painstaking production of an idealized persona, one marketed for mass consumption and artificial to a maximum degree. Those of us who inhabit the world outside the screen cannot compete with these apparent paragons and can only suffer by comparison. Our culture is growing to have an increasing intolerance for reality in all its manifold variety and imperfections. We can observe similar tendencies in the creation of an online avatar on social media, especially Facebook. The negative impact on self-esteem that obsessive involvement with Facebook engenders is well documented. It undoubtedly stems from the disconnect between real people's experience of their own flawed lives and their perception of others' artificial and faultless online personas.

The primary criterion for our assessment of a person seems ever more rooted in appearances,[1] in our embrace of visual aspects of their being, rather than qualities that might be considered more substantive, indicative of the soul that lies beyond the carefully crafted, manipulated visage.

Consistent with this visual hypertrophy, the elevation of the eye over the ear (see Chapter 4), a disturbing development has taken place in the world of classical vocalism. Studies have been conducted that demonstrate conclusively that winners of vocal competitions are increasingly being selected solely on the basis of how they look, not on the quality of the instrument itself. Participants in this research were shown only a video of the singers in a competition and asked to determine which performers were superior—without ever hearing their voices. Based on these criteria, they chose their favorites. The selection of the eventual winners by a panel of informed judges was shown to be markedly in alignment with the choices of persons who had no understanding of the intricacies of the art form and no direct experience of the crucial element—the singing voice.[2]

Many of the adjudicators in vocal competitions are professional singers themselves, for whom the beauty and expressiveness of the voice should be paramount. Despite this, in the study, they selected more physically appealing and recognizably emotive singers, due to the perception that because of their looks and marketability, they possess greater career potential, regardless of their native vocal talent or lack thereof.

One would presume that the art of Italianate *bel canto* (beautiful singing), some 500 years in its provenance, unlike contemporary popular music, would be resolutely impervious to the mainstream culture's single-minded fixation on looks. However, the stars who have risen to the top of the opera world in recent decades are markedly akin to their counterparts in the fields of popular entertainment. In our estimation, as professional singers who encountered colleagues from all over the world in our travels, these people do not *look* like opera singers; they more closely resemble musical theater singers or pop stars, and their voices are often less than remarkable. This phenomenon is not confined simply to the evaluation of singers; all professional creatives, regardless of genre, must now conform to society's expectations of attractiveness to achieve a degree of recognition in their fields.

This unremitting emphasis on the visual does great violence to individuals' self-images and has similarly produced a culture of "beauty" that regards the face as yet another fashion accessory to be modified at will, and, with the advent of whole-face transplants in the past few years, perhaps to be discarded in favor of next year's model.[3]

We have previously discussed the Yang nature of the eye, which subjects reality to its relentless and discriminatory gaze; however, the impartiality of the eye can be mitigated somewhat by a connection to the heart. Such is not the case with the icy cold regard of the camera lens or the iPhone screen.

Therefore, in electing to engage with the face for purposes of personal transformation, we seek to counteract the machinations of the visually driven beauty industry, which is mass-producing "individuals" who resemble nothing more than clones of some idealized somatotype or who, through the paralyzing agency of Botox, have transmogrified themselves in an extreme manner into emotionless androids.

The face is the most emotive, expressive part of the body; it has the capacity, through the agency of its intricate and subtle musculature, evolved through untold millennia, to reveal to the world the nature of our inner feeling life—to telegraph our joys, sorrows, anger, frustration, etc. In choosing to treat your patient's face, you are inviting them to undergo a ritual of authentic renewal, involving the release of emotions, which facilitates the connection to the heart, the repository of Shen. According to Chinese medicine, Shen is the radiance that emerges from the eyes, which expresses unconditional and nonjudgmental compassion.

Whether you are an acupuncturist, a complementary medicine professional, or a layperson, you will find that the capacity to share these treatments with your patients, family, or friends is a real gift; of course, it all depends upon how you receive that gift. This could be said about everything in life.

Vibrational Balancing Facial Protocol

1. Apply the Muse L'Herbal USA blended organic essential oil *Oil Essentiel Vert*, or one of the VibRadiance™ 5 Element Planetary

Essential Oil blends, mixed with our *Crème Vitale ESP Rose* (see Chapter 9), to the face and neck. Make sure that the patient is not allergic to any of the ingredients.

2. Have your patient, family member, friend, or loved one listen to and absorb the harmony of the Acutonics Ohm® Unison tuning forks prior to beginning the treatment. Then thoroughly ground them (see "The Grounding Protocol: A Vibratory Ritual of Earthing" in Chapter 8) with the tuning forks.

3. Activate the tuning forks by striking them on an Acutonics® belted acuvator (see "Tuning Forks" in Chapter 2 for instructions).

Specialized Techniques

◈ Holding: how you hold the tuning forks for this treatment is crucial. Prior to taking up the forks, ensure that you have thoroughly wiped your hands after massaging in the essential oil blend of your choice, mixed with the *Crème Vitale ESP Rose*. This will reduce the likelihood of you dropping one of the forks on the patient's face.

• Grasp the tuning forks by the yoke and strike them on the acuvator. Try to avoid making the extra "clinking" sound when doing so, and do not "attack" your patient's face. Approach the patient with a calm serenity; you are not going into battle.

As we've previously noted, the use of healing sound is an essentially Venusian treatment strategy, one that requires the development of a refined sense of "hearing" and the capacity, as a practitioner, both to be receptive in the moment and to restore receptivity. The ability to listen and respond is an increasingly marginalized faculty in our visual technocracy.

• Make sure that you are grounded, breathing into your Dantien, and practicing the tenets of Tai Chi—with circular, flowing, harmonious movement.

◈ Gliding: in this Ohm balancing facial, we will be *gliding* the forks up the neck, lubricated by the essential oil blend of your choice, and under the jaw and cheekbones to tone this area. We will not be lifting the forks off the face, but gently pinching, gliding, and moving—to the count of three.

❖ Sliding: to utilize this technique, it is essential to grasp the forks by the yoke, not the stem; the stem will be used to slide up and down the sides of the neck.

❖ Rolling: the stems of both forks will then be rolled behind and on either side of the back of the head, about 2 cun above the nape of the neck. Angle the stems bilaterally toward the center of the head.

Table 6.1 Instructions

Neck	Beginning at the clavicular notch, vibrate both forks on the clavicle, for three seconds. Then hold one Ohm fork on the clavicle and glide the other Ohm up the neck to the jawbone. Hold the second fork on the jawbone, just under the chin. Repeat the movements until the entire neck has been covered (resonated upon) once; hold each position for three seconds.
Chin	Gently pinch both Ohm forks together, using the stems on the jaw, one above and one below, to lift the area. Maintain each position for three seconds; treat bilaterally.
Smile line (nasolabial fold)	Vibrate both forks at the corner of the mouth (St-4 Dicang, Earth's Granary) for three seconds; then hold one Ohm at the corner of the mouth and glide the other perpendicularly up to the wing of the nose (LI-20 Yingxiang, Welcome Fragrance). Vibrate for three seconds; pinch the corner of the mouth and the wing of the nasolabial fold together vertically for three seconds. Treat bilaterally.
Cheekbones	From the wing of the nose (LI-20 Yingxiang) out to the ear, pinch, slide, and lift the cheekbones (zygomatic bone); place one fork under the bone and the other on top of the bone. Treat bilaterally and hold each position for three seconds.
Eyes	Vibrate both forks at the outer corner of the eye (GB-1 Tongziliao, Pupil Crevice); hold one fork on GB-1, then circle the other around the eye, in the direction that the eyebrow grows. Circle very gently and around each eyebrow three times; treat bilaterally.
Eyebrows	Pinch and lift the eyebrows, starting from the medial eyebrow (Bl-2 Zhanzhu, Gathered Bamboo) out to the lateral eyebrow (TH-23 Sizhukong, Silken Bamboo Hollow); hold each position for three seconds, and treat bilaterally.
Forehead	Cross-hatch the forehead: Glide the forks vertically, with one traveling up to the hairline and the other down to the brow; cover the entire area three times. Glide the forks horizontally from the center of the forehead out to the temples; treat each area three times (see Figure 6.1).

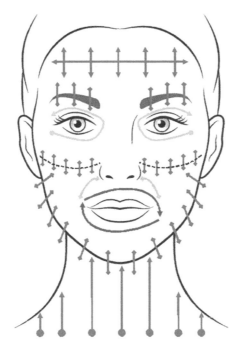

Figure 6.1 *The Vibrational Balancing Facial Protocol calms, relaxes, and grounds the patient*

Note: Lines with arrows indicate that the forks are to slide in the manner indicated; lines with diamonds at the end indicate a pinching action.

Treatment for the Platysma Muscle ("Turkey Wattles" or Sagging Neck)

The platysma, a long, quadrangular muscle, is the most superficial muscle of the face, and it produces transverse wrinkles in the skin of the neck. It is located in the fascia of the upper pectoralis and deltoideus muscles and extends the entire length of the neck to the angle of the mouth. This all-important muscle is so thin that a pathologist can easily peel it away prior to the further dissection of a cadaver. However, despite this seeming fragility, the platysma is a significant structural component of the facial musculature.

Table 6.2 The platysma muscle

Function	It contracts and pulls the corners of the mouth downward, raising the skin of the chest.
Emotions	Due to its function, the platysma is intimately involved with the expression of emotions such as grief, anxiety, suffering, and sadness. This is because its fibers interlace below the chin at the angle of the mouth. However, the platysma likewise has a role to play in the expression of happiness and joy when a person laughs or is feeling positive about their life.

We will be treating the platysma using motor points, both with acupuncture needling and tuning forks. To review, motor points are specific anatomical locations where nerves enter into muscles, otherwise known as neuromuscular junctions. When these sites are needled, or vibrated upon, the muscle fires, grabs the needle, and/or elicits a local twitch response. The status of the muscle, whether it is contracted or slack, is then relayed by the muscle spindle to the CNS, which then transmits instructions as to how the muscle may return to an optimal state of balance. Motor point treatments relax a tight muscle or strengthen a flaccid, weak muscle.

Follow the treatment diagram in Figure 6.2, starting with the chest area.

Table 6.3 The platysma: acupuncture needles

Treatment point #1	St-13 Qihu, Qi Door, is located under the clavicle, 4 cun laterally to the midline of the sternum.
Needling technique	Needle this point obliquely, laterally, and transversely, 0.3–0.5 cun outward toward the shoulders. Do not needle it perpendicularly, because deep needling can puncture the lung and could cause a pneumothorax.
	Use a Seirin #2 (0.18 gauge, 30 mm) to traverse this area under the clavicle. The needle should grab when pulled backward after needling; this is a motor point response.
Treatment point #2	"Blowfish" St-5 Daying, Great Welcome is an extra point located on top of the jaw, medial to TCM St-5 Daying and directly below St-4 Dicang, Earth's Granary.
	I refer to it as the "Blowfish" point because when patients are asked to puff out their cheeks, two distinct indentations appear.
Needling technique	Needle this point perpendicularly in the "Blowfish" indentation, then angle it horizontally outward along the jaw (see Figure 6.2). In order to confirm that you have needled the motor point correctly, pull back on it; it should grab and pucker the skin when you do so. There is usually not very much flesh in this area, so you do not need to insert the needle as deeply (0.2–0.3 cun). Needle bilaterally.

Treatment point #3	This point is just under extra point St-5 Daying, on the jawbone.
	This unusual technique is called "wrapping around the bone"; it uses one needle to access the jaw's attachment of muscles and tendons.
Needling technique	Palpate under extra point St-5 Daying on the jawline for an anatomical landmark, or indentation, in the jawbone. This is the site of the needle insertion; needle into this location, then angle the needle down toward the neck. Make sure that you have a sufficient length of needle under the skin so as to be able to literally wrap the needle down and around the bone. Needle bilaterally. Use a Seirin #2 (0.18 gauge, 30 mm) or a Seirin #3 (0.20 gauge, 30 mm) for thicker skin.

In needling these motor points, you may notice that a release of heat occurs at the insertion sites, and the patient's face may become quite red in the process. As the practitioner, you may likewise experience this release of heat, which is normal. I can recall several occasions when my own face became quite flushed during a demonstration of motor point needling, as did that of my assistant!

Tuning Fork Treatment for the Platysma Muscle

Table 6.4 The platysma: tuning forks

Treatment point #1	St-13 Qihu, Qi Door is located under the clavicle, 4 cun laterally to the midline of the sternum.
Tuning fork technique	Hold both Acutonics Ohm® Unison tuning forks on St-13, and resonate for three seconds. Then keep one fork on St-13 and glide the second fork 1 cun toward the shoulder. Hold the second fork in place, and allow the vibration to resonate between the two forks for three seconds.
Treatment point #2	Extra point St-5 Daying, Great Welcome is located on top of the jaw, medial to TCM St-5 Daying and directly below St-4 Dicang, Earth's Granary.
	When the patient puffs out their cheeks, two indentations appear on both sides of the jaw. These are the sites where you will position the tuning forks.
Tuning fork technique	Resonate both forks on "Blowfish" St-5 three times; then, while the first fork remains in place, move the other outward toward the ear, on top of the jaw, as shown in Figure 6.2 (about 1 cun).
	Please note: If the resonance is more readily absorbed on one side of the face than the other, this is indicative of a slackness or weakness on that side of the jaw. You may wish to treat the area a few more times.
Treatment point #3	This point is just under extra point St-5 Daying, on the jawbone.
	This innovative technique is called "wrapping around the bone"; you will be using tuning forks to traverse the same anatomical landscape as is engaged with the needling technique.

cont.

Tuning fork technique	Resonate the Acutonics Ohm® Unison tuning fork combination on the indentation on the jaw; apply the vibration to the area three times. Then hold one fork in position, and move the other down and around the jaw, angling out toward the ear, 1 cun. Repeat this procedure three times; treat bilaterally.

This vibrational protocol is very effective and can be incorporated into a sound treatment session.

Reminder: Do not use the acupuncture needling techniques for the platysma muscle if you are not a licensed acupuncturist (three-plus years of training).

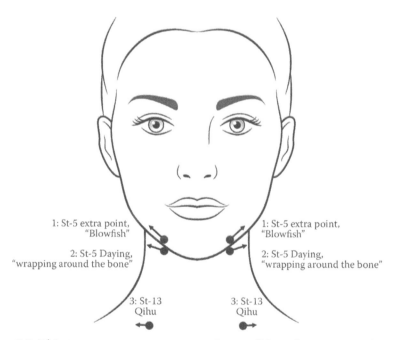

Figure 6.2 *This treatment uses motor points to lift and tone a sagging muscle*

Integrating the Two Modalities

Use the Acutonics Ohm® Unison tuning fork combination to activate the treatment points and then needle them; after you have done so, the motor points will be more responsive. The synergy of both Venus and Mars, Yin and Yang, produces a more dynamic result—gentle and powerful.

Chapter 7

~~~∞◦○◯○◦∞~~~

Vibrational Hara

All that we are is a result of what we have thought.

Buddha

This chapter introduces Five Element Japanese abdominal palpation and related treatments for specific syndromes. Noninvasive tuning fork treatments are stressed; however, instructions for acupuncture needling by itself, and the integration of the two relevant modalities, resonance and needling, will also be described.

Japanese diagnosis and abdominal treatments have been used for centuries to maintain health, well-being, and longevity.

Only staying active will make you want to live one hundred years.

Japanese proverb

According to Héctor García and Francesc Miralles, the authors of the book *Ikigai*, Japan has a high percentage of centenarians who are vibrant, active, and creative.[1] Everyone in Japan has *ikigai*—a reason for living—a spiritual calling or vocation. In fact, there is no Japanese expression that is the equivalent of the Western state of retirement. To them, happiness lies in the doing of a particular task, not in the results that one may achieve in the process thereof. Their extended life spans stem from a sense of community, a healthy diet, and the resilience that is part of their culture.

Fall seven times, rise up eight.

Japanese proverb

Wabi-sabi

The Japanese believe that beauty is imperfect and fleeting, whether it is a quality observed in an individual, a work of art such as Japanese pottery, *sogetsu* (Japanese flower arrangement), or heard in a piece of music. The concept of *wabi-sabi* embraces an awareness of impermanence, coupled with an understanding that everything changes. The moment only exists now: it will not return. This philosophy of "the moment" allows them to perpetually reinvent themselves and relinquish negative emotions and relationships that are no longer fruitful.

When I lived in Tokyo in the late 1980s, English was not spoken by the Japanese as much as it is at present, and there were no street signs in any language other than Japanese! Out of necessity, I learned to locate addresses and landmarks by recognizing familiar features in the city landscape; this was long before the advent and availability of global positioning systems (GPS)!

For example, I would memorize the following sequence of directions: "Turn right at the blue apartment building, go down the hill past the *koban* (police box or kiosk), and then continue straight for two streets. The hotel will be on the right side of the street."

The subways were, mercifully, color-coded, which allowed me to consult my English subway map, see the colors of the respective subway lines, and ascertain what my itinerary should be. This visual coding helped me find my way around the city, so that I could negotiate the hustle and bustle of Tokyo and her teeming masses of people.

I spent a great deal of time repeatedly getting lost, exploring neighborhoods that I might never have dreamed of visiting! These impromptu expeditions forced me to become conscious of every step I took. My linear, goal-oriented Western mind quieted for a while as I experienced a new world with fresh eyes.

This state of heightened intuitive sensitivity is echoed in a similar awareness and grounding cultivated by Japanese practitioners as they palpated their patients' haras, rhythmically following the flow of their inhalations and exhalations.

Japanese Hara Palpation

Palpation of the hara provides the practitioner with crucial information as to the general health of the patient's body, organs, and meridians. It also prepares the acu-sound points for treatment and functions as a preventative, harmonizing protocol.

According to Kiiko Matsumoto and her co-author Stephen Birch, palpation was used diagnostically in the Han Dynasty.[2] However, abdominal palpation and diagnosis developed very little thereafter in China, and few texts have much to say on this topic. Apparently, the Chinese were more reluctant to expose their abdomens to acupuncture physicians than the Japanese. Historically, Japanese society had much less in the way of inhibitions regarding public nudity.[3] They regularly visited the *onsen*, Japanese bathhouses, wearing their *yukata*, cotton robes, and *geta*, "sandals on stilts." For centuries, Japanese bathers had no compunctions about revealing their nude bodies to others, unashamedly unwrapping their *yukata* and lowering themselves into the baths for purposes of relaxation, health, and cleanliness.

When Chinese medicine was introduced to Japan in the early 5th century, Japanese practitioners found it easier to comprehend the Chinese texts by using palpation techniques.[4] Through the subsequent centuries, they refined these palpation skills and created a unique system of healing.

In the ancient text the *Nei Jing*, chapters NJ 15 and NJ 16, practitioners are provided with guidelines for abdominal palpation according to specific elements and the corresponding organ systems, as follows.[5]

- The sternum reflects the condition of the Heart and the Fire element; palpate below the sternum.

- The umbilicus relates to the Spleen and the Earth element; palpate around the umbilicus.

- The area below the umbilicus relates to the Kidney and the Water element; palpate below the umbilicus.

- The right side of the navel reflects the health of the Lung and the Metal element; palpate on the right side of the navel.

- The left side of the navel indicates imbalances in the Liver and the Wood element; palpate on the left side of the navel.

Guidelines

The practitioner's hands should be warmed before palpation begins, so as not to startle the patient. The practitioner must be calm, grounded, and composed as they begin the treatment. The abdomen embodies the source of Qi, and therefore, the *Nei Jing* stressed the importance of having the patient breathe properly during the palpation process.[6] According to the late Kuzome-sensei, a master shiatsu therapist in Japan, it is vital to synchronize hara palpation with the patient's breathing cycle. During treatments he would, to a count of six, apply perpendicular pressure with his fingertips to the Five Element areas of the hara.

Kuzome-sensei could detect any tight, tender, reactive abdominal areas, and to what regions of the body these sensations radiated. In so doing, he was able to ascertain which organs and elements were out of balance.[7]

Kuzome-Sensei's Six-Step Breathing Technique

1. As the patient inhaled, the practitioner would position his fingers and the hands over the abdomen.

2. The patient would then exhale, as the practitioner began to apply pressure to the count of one.

3. This exhalation would continue, and the pressure applied by the practitioner would increase to the count of two.

4. As the patient continued to expel their breath, a possible pain reaction, tenderness, or tightness could be discerned, to the count of three.

5. The patient continued the exhalation process, as the practitioner decreased the pressure to the count of four and then five.

6. With the end of the exhalation, the applied pressure was gradually released to the count of six.

The Wu Xing: The Five Elements

According to Chinese philosophy, the world is composed of five elements—Wood, Fire, Metal, Earth, and Water. These Five Elements are also referred to as the Five Phases, Five Movements, and Five Crossroads. According to Ted Kaptchuk, O.M.D., the usage of the term *element* rather than *phase* is a Western construct:

> The Chinese term we translate as "Five Phases" is Wu Xing. Wu is the number 5, and Xing means to "walk" or "move", implying a *process*. The Wu Xing, therefore, are five kinds of processes...a system of correspondences and patterns.[8]

> In ancient writings, *wu xing* meant crossroads. This more literal meaning had the symbolic advantage of implying the energetic coordinates of a larger astrological system.[9]

An ancient Chinese document referred to as the Ch'u Silk manuscript, discovered in 1942 in a tomb near Changsha, in Hunan province, and dating from c. 300 BCE (during the Han Dynasty), is the oldest surviving Chinese example of what might be termed an astro-calendrical almanac. The manuscript is arranged in the form of a calendar, depicting 12 figures considered to be the tutelary spirits of the individual months, i.e., the recognizable animals of the Chinese zodiac, and identifying, among other things, those associated with specific seasons.

Consistent with similar artifacts that relate to ancient cosmologies, the Ch'u Silk manuscript imparts crucial guidance as to how human beings can consciously align their activities with nature to promote a healthy flow of Qi. This established a harmony between the elements, the cycles of the seasons, the organs of the physical body, and colors as an extension of elemental correspondence. The information encoded in the Ch'u Silk manuscript is easily seen as relevant to many of the organizing principles of feng shui, and likewise is mirrored in the tenets of Chinese medicine, particularly in its Five Element theory.

The Five Elements have been utilized by the Chinese for centuries as a way of articulating humanity's implicit participation in the rhythms and structures of creation. By observing the action of these archetypal agencies in the manifestations of nature, for example, annual changes in rainfall, the force of the wind, etc., they could identify and predict the occurrence of related imbalances in the human body, thereby preventing illness and promoting longevity.

Five Element Correspondences

Each of the Five Elements was considered to relate to a range of archetypal phenomena, including a particular season, organ, color, sound, emotional state, etc. (as illustrated in Table 7.1):

Table 7.1 Five Element correspondence chart

Element	Wood	Fire	Earth	Metal	Water
Zang	Liver	Heart/Pericardium	Spleen	Lung	Kidney
Fu	Gall Bladder	Small Intestine/Triple Heater	Stomach	Large Intestine	Urinary Bladder
Sense	Sight	Speech	Taste	Smell	Hearing
Part nourished	Tendons	Vessels	Flesh	Skin	Bones
Flows to	Nails	Tongue	Mouth/lips	Body hair	Head hair
Fluid	Tears	Sweat	Saliva	Mucus	Urine
Smell	Rancid	Scorched	Fragrant	Rotten	Putrid
Emotion	Anger	Joy	Worry	Grief	Fear
Flavor	Sour	Bitter	Sweet	Pungent	Salty
Sound	Shouting	Laughing	Singing	Weeping	Groaning
Weather	Wind	Heat	Damp	Dry	Cold
Season	Spring	Summer	Late summer	Autumn	Winter
Color	Green	Red	Yellow	White	Blue/black
Direction	East	South	Central	West	North
Time	11pm–3am	7pm–11pm 11am–3pm	7am–11am	3am–7am	3pm–7pm
Spirit	Ethereal soul (Hun)	Mind (Shen)	Intellect (Yi)	Bodily soul (Po)	Will (Zhi)
Function	Smooth flow of Qi; stores blood	Houses Shen; circulates blood	Transforms and transports Qi; controls blood	Governs Qi and breathing; distributes Qi and body fluids	Controls Jing; stores water
Harmony	Motivated, organized, easygoing	Sensitive, joyful	Grounded, supportive, attentive, thoughtful	Positive communicator, vital	Determined, resourceful

Disharmony	Frustrated, angry, compulsive	Nervous, agitated, depressed, no self-esteem	Dependent, worried, overprotecting, self-doubt	Sad, pessimistic, remote	Insecure, driven, restless
Psychological	Motivated, adaptability	Awareness, harmony	Concentration, understanding	Boundaries, interactive, instinctive	Willpower, stamina, ingenuity
Expression	Compassion	Love	Empathy	Reverence	Wisdom

The Tao

To know harmony within and without is to be everlasting; to be everlasting is to obtain insight.

Tao Te Ching (chapter 55)

There is a well-established precedent in ancient documents to associate Chinese philosophy, politics, astrology, and cosmology with the Five Elements. The cyclical, transformational process embodied in this fivefold system of universal principles is seeded in the Chinese philosophy of the Tao.

The Tao is the organizing agency implicit in the manifold processes of nature—how life force is created, sustained, and changes through time. This perspective evolved out of observing the natural order as embodied in the cycles of the seasons. It is wholeness stemming from a dynamic equilibrium that consists of interacting opposites spawning each other. Every life unfolds in accordance with the perpetual cycles of birth, growth, ripening, decline, and death. No organic life-form can escape the dictates of these natural developmental stages that mirror nature and the ongoing evolutionary movement that occurs with each passing season.

Yin and Yang

Out of the Tao come Yin and Yang—complementary opposites that together encompass in their purview all aspects of life and matter.

Table 7.2 Yin and Yang

Yin	Yang
Night	Day
Passive	Active
Stillness	Movement
Cold	Hot
Water	Fire
Moist	Dry
Emotional	Logical
Intuitive	Intellectual
Acceptance	Willfulness
Earth	Heaven
Peaceful	Violent
Invisible	Visible
Form	Function
Dense	Gaseous
Nurturing	Consuming
Inner	Outer
Contracting	Expanding
Downward	Upward

This twofold conception of the Yin and Yang establishes a structural paradigm for the physical universe in which the interrelationship, and continual transmutation, of these two fundamental principles engenders the infinite manifestations of matter and spirit. The energy that powers this unceasing process of cosmic evolution is embodied in the pivotal conception of Qi.

Qi (Chi)

Qi is the life force and cosmological glue that inextricably binds Yin and Yang—interacting, flowing, opposing, and balancing each other. The Chinese character for Qi depicts steam rising over rice, which symbolically provides nourishment, and simply translated, Qi means "breath." Specifically, this breath of life nourishes and animates all things, not merely organic life—animals, fish, flowers, and trees, but also rocks, to the entire order of creation all the way to its pinnacle, humanity. Qi gives rise to nature in all its myriad splendor—mountains, rivers, plants—and is the unifying life force that links all living things.

Qi animates our bodies, our intellectual processes, and speech, and sparks our Shen spirit. It connects us to our true self, which swims in the primordial, cosmological amniotic fluid, awaiting the hour of its arrival on the earth plane. This primal force propels us in our journey from birth to death, equipping us with the wisdom and insight to recognize loved ones as they age by the radiance of their Shen spirit and the luminescence that reveals itself in their eyes.

The Five Elements as a "Crossroads"

The intersection and intermingling of Wood, Fire, Earth, Metal, and Water can be observed in the infinite variety of natural phenomena, which is the natural world in perpetual motion and change. In accordance with an ancient paradigm, the elements are in a dynamic process of transformation from one state to another: Wood grows and flourishes; Fire is hot and flares up; Earth is the center, and the progenitor, of all things; Metal descends and is clear; Water is cold and flows downward.

These cycles further explain the movement of Qi within the body, as it is transported throughout various organ systems designated as the Zang-Fu. Yin organs are identified as Zang, for example, the Liver, and Yang organs are Fu, such as the Gall Bladder. The cycles also form a relationship to one another, to humans, to the material world, and to the cosmos. The ebb and flow of Qi within the microcosm of the human body is yet another expression of the cyclical processes found throughout the universe.

A comprehension of the underlying movement of this vital force, through a reading of these elemental signposts, is essential to the process of diagnosis and treatment of constitutional imbalance and Qi disturbance that may affect a patient.

The Creative (Sheng) Cycle

This sequence promotes and supports growth and well-being. In this elemental cycle:

- Wood burns and promotes Fire; in the presence of Fire, Wood ignites, feeds the Fire, and is ultimately consumed by it

- the ash remaining from the Fire creates Earth; the remains of the burned Wood are deposited on the ground as ashes and become a part of the soil

- Earth's minerals become Metal; the veins of raw minerals found deep within the earth are extracted by various means and chemically transformed to produce Metal

- through condensation and melting, Metal becomes Water

- Water flows freely on the surface of, and within, the ground, and nourishes plant and animal life, including trees, the embodiment of the Wood element.

This cycle begins anew in a timeless loop, and human beings participate in this eternal flow of element to element, witnessing the process in the cycles of the seasons and in their own personal development.

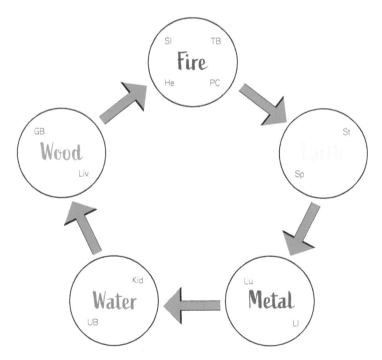

Figure 7.1 *The keyword in this creative cycle is promoting; the previous element generates and promotes the next in a normal energetic relationship*

Wood Promotes Fire

If the mother (Wood) is unable to support or feed her child (Fire), then she needs help from her own mother, Water, the previous element of the cycle. We can draw an analogy here to the guidelines imparted by the flight crews on major airlines concerning the proper procedures for dealing with a lack of oxygen in the cabin, i.e., the mother must put on her oxygen mask first and then assist her child. If she lapses into unconsciousness because of a lack of oxygen and cannot see to her child's needs, there is an increased probability that the child will not survive.

The Controlling (Ko) Cycle

This contrary cycle balances and coordinates the elements during times of change and growth. Within it, the elements interact in a manner that is detrimental to their optimal functioning, and this can contribute to constitutional imbalance. However, the limitations imposed upon other elements by those that are in control of them, their checking aspects, serve to ensure that no one element becomes excess or hyperactive.

Some examples are given below.

⬦ Metal, in the form of an ax or saw, cuts Wood. Metal is the agency by which the life of a tree is prematurely cut short, so that its Wood may be harvested.

⬦ Wood destroys Earth. A tree thrusts its roots deep into the Earth, breaking up the integrity of the soil, while also leaching the ground of vital nutrients.

⬦ Earth, in the form of an earthen dike, absorbs Water. Water that falls upon the ground is readily absorbed and cannot flow freely and easily.

⬦ Water extinguishes Fire. A Fire is deprived of oxygen and snuffed out when it is inundated by Water.

⬦ Fire can scorch and melt Metal. A sufficiently hot flame will destroy the structural integrity of Metal, causing it to flow like a liquid.

An excess of one of the elements will contribute to that element overacting on the weaker elements. This may give rise to certain pathologies.

For example: if Earth, which relates to the Zang-Fu pairing of Spleen/Stomach, is weak or deficient, and the Wood, Liver/Gall Bladder, is strong or excess, the Liver could overact on the Spleen. This imbalance can contribute to the development of irritable bowel syndrome (IBS), related digestive problems, and a lack of grounding, among other syndromes.

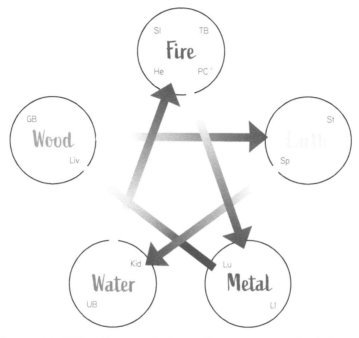

Figure 7.2 *If the Liver pathologically overacts on the Spleen, it can cause digestive problems, such as IBS, acid reflux, etc.*

A third, pathological phase is designated as counteracting. This cycle is the opposite of the overacting "Ko" cycle. Ordinarily, Metal acts on Wood, but if Wood is hyperactive and Metal is deficient, Wood could counteract on Metal, causing a hyperactive diaphragm and breathing difficulties.

Japanese Five Element Hara Treatments

Table 7.1 provides a comprehensive catalog of correspondences for each of the Five Elements, ranging from the relevant Zang-Fu organs to color, flavor, smell, season, etc., as well as psychospiritual imbalances that may result in various pathologies.

Also included in this chapter are Japanese hara palpation techniques for each element and treatment protocols for addressing various syndromes with tuning forks and/or acupuncture needles. If you wish to learn more Japanese treatments for the Five Elements, please consult Chapter 4 of Mary Elizabeth's book *Constitutional Facial Acupuncture*.[10]

A clinical note: I strongly recommend using sound in the following elemental treatments. If you are not a licensed or registered acupuncturist and have not trained for three-plus years in an accredited school, do not attempt to insert acupuncture needles into yourself or another person. You may cause harm, and this could subject you to accusations of malpractice and possible legal ramifications.

Wood Element

Hun: the Ethereal Soul

This soul represents the Spirit of the Liver. The ancient Chinese believed that when the body, the corporeal soul, died, the eternal Hun spirit would eventually reincarnate and continue its journey in a new form.

While embodied in a given incarnation, the Hun is a source of guidance, inspiration, purpose, happiness, and transformative experiences. Blockages in the Liver may contribute to states of depression, disorientation, and disconnection from the soul (Hun).

The Wood Element Personality

As you will have observed, each of the Five Elements can become either excess or deficient, giving rise to certain polarized extremes of personality and behavior. When the Wood element is balanced, the person is flexible, creative, motivated, adaptable, and easygoing. When out of balance, they are ungrounded, frustrated, angry, and compulsive, and have difficulty making a decision.

The Liver excels in strategic planning and, functionally, it stores and regulates blood, harmonizes emotions, and rules the flow of Qi throughout the body. The Gall Bladder, its Yang partner, excels in making decisions and judgments; functionally, it stores and excretes bile to aid in digestion.

Wood Element Imbalances

Liver and Gall Bladder imbalances can be more pronounced on the right side of the body. The person may have weight issues, hepatitis, cirrhosis of the liver, a fatty liver, or addictions to alcohol or drugs such as prescription pain relievers, including opioids, for example, fentanyl, Vicodin, Percodan, Percocet. They could also have migraines, hormonal headaches, tendinomuscular spasms, tics, and TMJ. According to Chinese medicine, the state of depression is a manifestation of a disharmonious Liver.

The Wood element person may also have allergies to certain cosmetics and creams, a sensitivity to insect bites, and seasonal allergies, especially in the springtime, the season of Wood. As the Liver is responsible for moving Qi and blood, systemic blood stagnation may result when this function is blocked, imbalanced, or otherwise compromised.

The Japanese refer to this syndrome as *oketsu*, which means "stuck blood." When blood is stagnant, masses may develop in the body, such as uterine fibroids and cystic breasts. *Oketsu* can be attributed to:

⊕ blood transfusions after surgery

⊕ scars that may develop in the aftermath of surgery or injuries resulting from accidents

⊕ right-side occipital pain and headache

⊕ PMS

⊕ dark circles under the eyes related to the Liver

⊕ depression, anger, frustration.

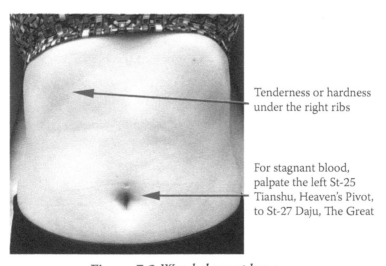

Tenderness or hardness under the right ribs

For stagnant blood, palpate the left St-25 Tianshu, Heaven's Pivot, to St-27 Daju, The Great

Figure 7.3 *Wood element hara*

Japanese Oketsu Hara Palpation

> Please note: Palpation of the hara is for diagnostic purposes only.

The Liver hara is only palpated on the left side of the navel from St-25 Tianshu to St-27 Daju, and under the right rib cage. This is because the mesenteric and hepatic portal veins flow from the left side of the hara and up to the Liver organ to cleanse toxic blood. It may also be why the Liver pulse is palpated on the left side of the wrist. For those of you who are non-acupuncturists, the width of a person's thumb is considered to be a "human inch," or a cun. (See Figure 7.3.)

Follow Kuzome-sensei's instructions for hara palpation (see "Guidelines" earlier in this chapter) and feel for tight, tender, sensitive areas on the left side of the navel and under the right rib cage. If there is tightness, and the person has recently been operated upon, has a preexisting scar, or is suffering from PMS or a headache with pain concentrated behind the eyes, they will undoubtedly benefit from the treatment for the Wood element hara.

Japanese Oketsu; Stuck Blood

Location: palpate the left abdominal area only, 2 cun out from the navel, and 2 cun down from the navel. Look for any tightness or tenderness.

If this area is tight, treat the body on the left side only.

Treatment points:

1. Japanese Lu-5 Chize, Cubit Marsh; when the forearm is palm up, the point is in the crease of the elbow on the thumb side of the arm. It is located on the cubital crease of the elbow, midway between TCM Lu-5 Chize and TCM LI-11 Quchi, Pool at the Crook. The point is found 1 cun above or below this area. Angle the acupuncture needles or Acutonics Ohm® Unison tuning forks down toward the feet for Japanese Lu-5 Chize, and up toward the head for TCM Liv-4 Zhongfeng. This follows the flow of Qi in the meridians.

2. Japanese Liv 4 Zhongfeng, Middle Seal; 1 cun from the inner ankle bone. It is lateral to the medial malleolus, midway between TCM Sp-5 Shangqui, Shang Mound, and TCM St-41 Jiezi, Middle Seal, in the depression on the medial side of the tibialis anterior tendon.[11]

For emotional stress, anger, tightness, spasms, chronic headaches, menstrual cramps, PMS, cystic breasts, dark circles under the eyes, and irritability, vibrate the Acutonics Ohm® Unison tuning forks on, or insert two Seirin #1 (0.16 gauge, 30 mm) needles into, these points.

Tuning Forks vs. Needles: Recommendations

Once again, using tuning forks for the vibrational hara protocols instead of needles is highly recommended. The Acutonics Ohm® Unison tuning fork combination instills a sense of calm, and the forks' Earth vibration is highly effective for grounding and balancing a patient. When resonated simultaneously, they engender a musical interval, the Ohm Unison, which, as we learned in Chapter 1, can be likened to the undifferentiated perfection of the universe in the moments before the Big Bang.

The tone Ohm specifically relates to Earth, due to its mathematical derivation, according to the formula established by Hans Cousto in *The Cosmic Octave*, from the duration of our planet's orbital cycle around the Sun every year: "The length of time a celestial body takes to…revolve around the sun can be converted to sound…by means of the law of the octave. These sounds…are analogous to that which presents itself in the heavens."[12]

This synergy of harmonious interval and elemental Earth further enhances the grounding potency of this tuning fork combination, which can be a palliative for technology-addicted, overstressed, excessively Yang individuals. It introduces them to a component of Yin receptivity that is becoming altogether too rare in our pathologically Yang culture.

In the Introduction, we alluded to the concept of balanced, harmonious music in ancient China, which also linked humanity to the twin realms of the cosmos and Earth, making it theoretically possible for human beings to experience the entirety of what the Chinese refer to as the Three Treasures: Heaven, Earth, and Humanity. In this tripartite conception of the physical universe, humanity inhabits the middle ground between Heaven (cosmos) and Earth. Grounding and centering your patients with these planetary tuning forks is very much in alignment with this ancient notion of exposure to upright music, as well as with Pythagorean philosophy, which stressed the importance of humans being attuned to cosmic resonance.

Sound is transmitted four times faster through water than air, and it has the capacity to reach every cell of the body because of the predominantly aqueous constituency of our tissues and organs, as well as the body's highly conductive skeletal framework. Additionally, each cell contains within its cellular membrane highly specialized proteins called aquaporins, or "water channel" proteins, that facilitate the transmission of water across that boundary. The marrow of our bones is Kidney essence and, therefore, healing sound can harmonize our bodies at their very core.

Sound as an Adaptogen

The use of the Acutonics Ohm® tuning forks restores the body's natural balance without the risk of overtreating the patient. In other words, sound vibration adapts itself to the needs of the person being treated. This is because you, as the practitioner, participate in a feedback loop, i.e., if you feel the sound vibrations traveling up your arm, your patient's body has absorbed the resonance it required, and you are now the recipient of a treatment you do not necessarily need. Don't fork further! Move on to the next set of points, or conclude the treatment, as is appropriate.

By way of contrast, acupuncture, microcurrent, and other modalities are subject to overtreatment, and overtreatment is like overeating—it can become an addiction! The following section presents an interesting example of this type of addiction.

A Galvanic Current Junkie

I had a patient who, curiously enough, had developed an addiction to galvanic current, as administered by an esthetician, to keep her face lifted and toned. Galvanic spa machines charge the skin with a low-voltage DC current via a conductive treatment gel applied prior to the treatment by the practitioner.

In this instance, she had been receiving this treatment every week for 15 years. On those occasions when she failed to receive her weekly dose of "juice," her subjective impression was that her skin suffered as a result, appearing rather more saggy than she ideally would have wished. However, she was beginning to have headaches and felt that she was very dependent on these treatments. She sounded me out about the possibility of receiving tuning fork facial treatments, a vibrational protocol we refer to as *Facial Soundscapes*™.[13]

When I gave her a tuning fork treatment that addressed both constitutional and facial treatment points, it seemed to eliminate the headaches. She also observed that her face "lifted" dramatically. However, after a few sessions, she remarked that, in her opinion, the results of these vibrational treatments did not hold as long as the galvanic current sessions. She also further observed that she seemed to be experiencing a detox from the electricity that was both physical and emotional in impact.

After only four sessions, she informed me that she no longer wished to continue with the tuning fork treatments, because she was emotionally dependent upon the electricity. She admitted that she was addicted and was unwilling to continue with the sound therapy, because she didn't wish to experience any withdrawal symptoms.

This is indeed a peculiar story... The vibrational treatments evoked an unaccustomed receptivity in her and a necessity for patience with the gradual nature of the process. She lacked the perseverance to continue with this modality and wanted a "quick fix." The galvanic current undoubtedly provided a stimulating effect that was in direct contrast to the sedating and tranquilizing nature of the vibrational protocols. This is something that you will need to consider when you are working with healing sound.

Treatments with modalities such as galvanic current are effective because they address the electrical aspect of our being. Our nervous system transmits information by means of minute electrochemical reactions, through the interaction and exchange of potassium and sodium ions; however, vibrational therapies are potentially more transformative in their effects. They do not feed into the overwhelmingly electrical paradigm that increasingly informs our world; we are still discovering what the cumulative deleterious effects of continuous exposure to electricity and microwaves might be. Vibrational healing modalities permit us to switch off, returning to a more organic and harmonious way of being. My "electro-junkie" patient, on the other hand, would not permit herself to be unplugged from the mains. She switched back to electricity, the headaches resumed, and her addiction continued unchecked.

Fire Element

Shen: the Compassionate Soul

The Shen Spirit is the immortal spirit essence that enlivens physical existence in successive incarnations. It is our spiritual center, and the light that shines forth from our eyes and connects us to our heart's compassion. The radiance of Shen emerges from deep within our being and sheds its light upon the material world and those around us; it vividly attests to the spiritual fire that is embodied in our true natures. Shen emanates from understanding and unconditional love. An individual with an underactive heart center, who has lost this vital connection to their Shen, housed in the physical heart, can suffer a profound loss of spiritual identity.

The Fire Element Personality

A Fire element person is passionate, exciting, dynamic, and vibrant. Fire ascends heavenward, lifts the spirit, and is linked to the Sun's life-giving rays, which unconditionally provide warmth and light to humanity. The living embodiment of this element is the great ball of fire at the heart of our solar system, the Sun, which, in a perpetual act of altruism and self-immolation, provides the light and energy that sustains our entire ecosystem.

In the *Nei Jing*, the Heart is described as the monarch, who excels in thought, insight, and understanding. Functionally, the Heart controls and circulates blood, and houses the Shen spirit. The Small Intestine receives and transforms food and separates the pure from the impure, including unnecessary thoughts and emotions.

Both the Pericardium and the Triple Heater (Burner) do not house organs; however, their functions are very important in Chinese medicine. The Pericardium is called the Heart Protector, because it wraps around the Heart and guards the heart muscle from shock or trauma.

The Pericardium meridian is also called Circulation Sex. In the *Nei Jing*, it is described as the official who guides the subjects in the joys and pleasures by encouraging blood flow, the production of sexual fluids, balanced Shen, and relationship.

The Triple Heater (Burner) has an important and mystical function in Chinese medicine. The ancient Taoists used alchemical practices to transform the Three Jiaos via meditation, breathing techniques, and ingestion of minerals and substances to transform the Three Treasures— Jing, Qi, and Shen.

Fire Element Imbalances

Heart disease may be inherited from the family and manifest as symptoms such as palpitations, high or low blood pressure (hyper-/hypotension), mitral valve prolapse, rheumatic fever, or pericarditis. A Fire person tends to be a Type A personality, one who is usually subject to a great deal of stress, the symptoms of which may be anxiety, restlessness, nervousness, and insomnia.

If a patient presents with cardiac issues, it is important not to treat the area over the heart, but to bring the Qi down to the feet, away from the heart organ. Treating a patient locally in this fashion, with Acutonics Ohm® Unison tuning forks or acupuncture needles, may exacerbate their condition.

The following section includes two Japanese treatments for Heart imbalances.

The treatment for palpitations:

◈ alleviates anxiety

◈ relaxes the pulse

◈ soothes the heartbeat.

Contraindications: If a patient has a pacemaker or a slow pulse, do not treat these points.

The treatment for high or low blood pressure (hyper- or hypotension) and shortness of breath:

- homeostatically regulates both high and low blood pressure

- opens the chest and helps the patient to breathe with greater ease

- treats shortness of breath and "white coat" syndrome

- addresses both lethargy and cold sensations (hypotension) and anxiety and Heart heat (hypertension).

Please note that these points help to calm patients who are subject to "white coat syndrome," i.e., fear of the physician. Doctors have a regrettable tendency to unilaterally prescribe blood pressure medication for all patients once they reach a certain age, without taking individual needs into consideration. Generalized anxiety and sheer dread of the possibility of an adverse diagnosis by the physician quickens these patients' breathing, which can cause the pulse to race. Treating the indicated points with acu-sound therapy, instructing the patient as to the importance of deep abdominal breathing, and helping them visualize a beautiful, unstressful place usually relaxes the pulse. If the patient is legitimately in need of medication, they will receive it.

Japanese Fire Element Hara Palpation

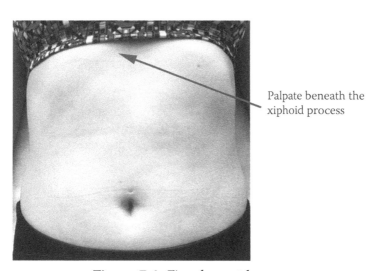

Palpate beneath the xiphoid process

Figure 7.4 *Fire element hara*

Palpate the hara with one hand placed atop the other, up toward the xiphoid process; palpate 45 degrees upward, just under the sternum.

Feel for tight, tender points, sensitivity, or localized pain. The patient who complains of palpitations, hypertension, or stress may exhibit an intense pulse below the xiphoid process, just under the rib cage.

Japanese Treatment Points for Palpitations

Vibrate the Acutonics Ohm® Unison tuning forks, or insert two Seirin #1 (0.16 gauge 15 mm) acupuncture needles bilaterally, or needle/fork perpendicularly, in the middle of the crease behind the second toe for palpitations, fast heartbeat, or irregular heartbeat.

> Contraindications: Do not treat these points if there is a slow pulse or the patient has a pacemaker.

Japanese Treatment Points for Blood Pressure and Shortness of Breath

Vibrate the Acutonics Ohm® Unison tuning fork combination, or insert two Seirin #1 (0.16 gauge 15 mm) acupuncture needles bilaterally, behind the third toe, in the middle of the crease where the sole of the foot meets the toe. However, the noninvasive tuning forks are recommended.

Other recommendations: For palpitations, blood pressure imbalances, and shortness of breath, apply 800 gauss non-gold-plated magnets to these points to provide support for the patient when they visit the doctor.

Earth Element
Yi: The Intellect

Yi, the Intellect, is an acquired part of the soul that relates to consciousness, awareness, and thought.

The Earth Element Personality

Earth represents our center, our grounding, and our home. It regulates all the cycles in our lives—from sleeping, breathing, and thinking, to the menstrual cycle. Earth is the source of physical nourishment and roots us in our bodies.

A person who is in harmony with the Earth is grounded, centered, attentive, thoughtful, and at home with themselves and the world. If imbalanced, they can be codependent, obsessed, uprooted, worried, and searching for support or answers outside themselves. An excess of the Earth element produces an overintellectual temperament, while those individuals with deficient Earth cannot process information.

The emotional expression of Earth in an imbalanced state manifests as a constant need for sympathy or an inability to receive any kind of emotional support in troubled times. A balanced state embraces empathy and compassion, while the individual remains centered in their Qi.

Earth Element Imbalances

Spleen and Stomach imbalances are more pronounced on the left side of the body where the actual organs are housed. The consumption of fast foods or genetically modified (GMO) foods, coupled with ever-increasing levels of stress, fosters blood sugar imbalances, i.e., hypoglycemia and diabetes, which affect the brain. Patients are unable to concentrate or think clearly, and symptoms are better or worse with, or without, food; before a meal, they may develop a headache or feel irritable or shaky. After eating, they usually fall asleep.

Even though there is a desire to lose weight, these individuals have developed poor, irregular eating habits; they are subject to food cravings and lack the willpower to change their diet and lifestyle. Due to blood sugar issues and hindered flow of oxygen, there can be cramping in the muscle tissues, e.g., the calf muscles, and the abdomen may be very sensitive and ticklish.

Sometimes, the immune system is compromised by food allergies, parasites, candida, and bacteria in the gut. In Chinese medicine theory, the Spleen holds the blood in the vessels and, when this function is impaired, irregular menses and excessive bleeding may develop. Bunions, which develop on the Spleen side of the big toe, in the Sp-3 Taibai, Supreme White, area, are also indicative of Earth element disharmony.

The Spleen Qi lifts the organs, and when it is deficient, there may be prolapses of the uterus, vagina, bladder, and anus. The Spleen also regulates fluids; deficiency may likewise produce symptoms such as puffiness of the inner canthus of the eye, and edema in the medial knee area, legs, and ankles.

Symptoms include:

- dizziness

- palpitations

- swollen ankles, medial knees, and the inner canthus of the eye

- gas and bloating

- stress

- prolapses

- shoulder and neck pain

- tension headaches.

Japanese Earth Element Hara Palpation

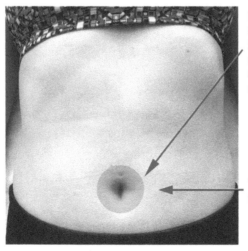

Palpate around the navel, and notice any cold sensations in that area; note, as well, any tension under the left rib cage and at the top of the shoulders

Tightness and pain around the navel area

Figure 7.5 *Earth element hara*

Location: palpate all around the navel; make a note of any nodules, sensitivity, or pain. Also palpate the tops of the shoulders (trapezius muscle) for tightness caused by stress, a weak Spleen, and lack of grounding.

If these areas are tight, treat Sp-9 Yinlingquan, bilaterally on the inside of the lower leg, in the depression under the knee.

Diagnostic Discernment

In order to discern whether the shoulders manifest a deficiency tightness, palpate GB-21 Jianjing, Shoulder Well, on the top of the shoulders/trapezius muscle. If the shoulders are indeed tense and tight, hold Sp-9 Yinlingquan, Yin Mound Spring, bilaterally for 30 seconds, pressing upward with your thumbs toward the shoulders.

Then recheck the condition of the shoulders, to see if they feel more relaxed. If they are softer, treat then with acupuncture needles, Acutonics Ohm® Unison tuning forks, or both modalities simultaneously.

Treatment Points for Deficiency-Related Tightness in the Shoulders

Sp-9 Yinlingquan is located on the medial side of the lower leg, in a depression in the angle formed by the medial condyle of the tibia and the posterior border of the tibia. It is a He-Sea Water point, which is the most important point on the Spleen meridian to alleviate the accumulation of damp fluid in the area of the knee, ankles, and inner canthus of the eye, and for tight shoulder muscles.

For very tight shoulders, resonate the Acutonics® Low Ohm Unison tuning forks on Sp-9 Yinlingquan, angled upward toward the shoulders, three times. If the resonance fades quickly, reactivate the tuning fork combination once again until the resonance holds longer. This indicates that the patient is not absorbing the frequency as readily and the Earth element is deficient. Following this procedure, check to see if the shoulders have become softer.

You may also insert Seirin #5 (0.25 gauge, 40 mm) acupuncture needles horizontally and angled upward from Sp-9 Yinlingquan toward GB-21 Jianjing. The intention of this treatment is to support and strengthen the Spleen, Earth element, and to likewise address conditions such as IBS, other digestive complaints, and a lack of grounding.

Metal Element

Po: The Corporeal Soul

The Po is the bodily soul that exists only for the duration of the life of the physical body. The body protects us, makes us aware of danger, and serves as a source of vitality and strength. The comparative fragility of our bodies causes us to be highly attuned to threats in our physical environment, which invests us with an appropriate caution. The Po is a reflection of our animal passion, the vehicle for the expression of our instinctual level of existence, those innate drives that have permitted us to survive as a species.

Our first breath would not be possible without the Lung. Breath is the medium for our verbal communication with others and, consequently, it facilitates the development of relationship.

The Metal Element Personality

The Lung takes in Qi and breath, while its Yang partner, the Large Intestine, eliminates unwanted substances from the body. When a Metal element person is balanced, they are positive and communicative, and have abundant Qi and energy. When imbalanced, they are sad, pessimistic, and remote.

The Lung is the only organ that connects us to the inner and outer worlds of Heaven, Tian, and Earth, Tu. Taking in a breath, "inspiration," links us to heavenly Qi, creativity, and vibrancy, while letting go and releasing the breath, "expiration," connects us again to Earth. We, humanity, inhabit the middle ground between Earth and Heaven, and possess the capacity within ourselves to reach for the stars while still rooted in the soil of our beautiful planet. According to the ancient Chinese, this dual process of breathing in vitality and relinquishing the old engenders reverence and simplicity.

Metal Element Imbalances

The Lung rules protective Wei Qi and the functioning of the immune system. Patients with poor immune systems are prone to catch colds and flu and are unable to recover from these upper respiratory illnesses with any alacrity.

According to Japanese acupuncture, a previous tonsillectomy negatively impacts the immune system. Weak connective tissue also relates to the vitality of a patient's immune response, and likewise to loose ligaments and collagen disorder.

The Metal element complexion tends to be pale, delicate, dry, and prone to wrinkles and sagging. Large Intestine imbalances manifest as constipation, diarrhea, sinus infections, and nasal discharge.

Symptoms include:

◈ tendonitis of the elbow

◈ sprained ankles

◈ a weak patellar ligament of the knee

◈ swollen lymph glands

◈ low immunity, lassitude, and fatigue

◈ a compromised immune system.

Japanese Metal Element Hara Palpation

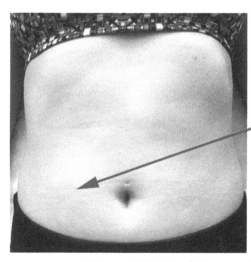

Palpate the right St-25 Tianshu, Heaven's Pivot, to St-27 Daju, The Great

Figure 7.6 *Metal element hara*

The Metal element hara is palpated in the same area as the Wood element hara, only on the right side of the abdomen. Once again, palpate St-25 Tianshu, Heaven's Pivot, down to St-27 Daju, The Great.

Look for a feeling of tightness or tenderness or a referred pain reaction in the abdomen. If your patient experiences these sensations, treat the Metal element.

Location: palpate the right abdominal area, 2 cun out from the navel, and 2 cun down from the navel.

If this area is tight, treat bilaterally: Japanese T.I. 10; locate by bending the arm inward toward the solar plexus. The point is below the elbow crease, toward the outer portion of the elbow.

Japanese Treatment for Immune Deficiency

The Japanese point for tonifying the immune system is called Triple Intestine 10 by Matsumoto-sensei. The innovative name for this point derives from its position between the Large Intestine and Triple Heater (Burner) meridians. It is very effective in the treatment of tennis elbow, tendonitis due to repetitive strain, and sports injuries. It is also used as a tonification point to address immune deficiency. The Japanese have observed, as noted above, that weak connective tissue relates to the health of the immune system.

Japanese Triple Intestine 10 (T.I. 10) is located between TCM LI-10 Shousanli, Arm Three Miles, and TCM LI-11 Quchi, Pool at the Crook. TCM LI-11 Quchi is in the depression at the end of the elbow crease, when the hand is placed on the chest. TCM LI-10 Shousanli is 2 cun below TCM LI-11 Quchi. The immune point is halfway between these two points.

Needling technique: Insert the acupuncture needle 90 degrees and angle it toward the bone and the Triple Heater meridian. Make sure that the patient's elbows are bent and placed over their solar plexus, with the palms facing the body. First, palpate this area cross-fiber to discern where to place the needles. The supinator muscle is usually involved in tennis elbow. It is the primary supinator of the hand and forearm and the radioulnar joint of the forearm. Symptoms may occur when a tennis player hits the ball off center, in a backhand stroke. Use a Seirin #1 (0.16 gauge, 30 mm) needle, angled toward the bone, bilaterally.

Tuning forks: Angle the Acutonics Ohm® Unison tuning forks toward the bone, and vibrate them three times. You can choose to place the two tuning forks on the affected tennis elbow side, or position one on each elbow to balance the immune system.

As previously noted, sound is adaptogenic in nature, and if you are in the general area, the resonance will travel to where it is needed. In palpating this area, you may feel multiple knots and tensions. Treat the area that is most tender.

Once again, remember that low immunity has a negative effect on connective tissue, which is comprised of ligaments and collagen-elastin fibers. When an avid tennis player complains of tennis elbow/tendonitis, they may also have immune deficiency imbalance.

Tuning forks and acupuncture needles: You can integrate tuning forks and acupuncture needles for a patient who is experiencing local pain in the elbow and for immune-system-related syndromes, such as colds, flu, and bronchitis. Needle the points first and then use the tuning forks around the needles. This treatment is also effective for patients who have chronic immune deficiency and/or an acute onset of a cold, flu, or bronchitis.

Forks: Acutonics Ohm® Unison Combination

Clinical note: Connective tissue supports, binds, and separates the organs and tissues of the body. Fibroblast cells produce connective tissue and are the precursors to collagen and elastin production. Japanese doctors agree that weak tendons and ligaments arise in the wake of focal infections in the sinuses, which compromise the immune system.

Water Element
Zhi: Willpower

The Spirit soul of the Water Element is the will, which is the basis of our endurance, determination, and perseverance. It gives us the drive and ability to accomplish tasks and to realize creative inspirations, dreams, and ambitions in life. A weak-willed person may have difficulty achieving their goals, because a deficiency in the Water element results in the reduction of drive and diminished willpower.

The Water Element Personality

Water assumes the shape of every container, and over time wears away anything in its path, from a pebble to a rock, or a boulder, or a large sequoia tree. It is fluid and flows either gently and peacefully or violently and powerfully.

It is paramount for life. The adult body is comprised of 70–78 percent water, which includes lymphatic fluid, saliva, and synovial fluid. We float effortlessly in the timeless watery sea of the womb while we are *in utero*, throughout the entirety of the nine-month gestation period prior to birth. My spiritual teacher, Dr. Beverly Lanzetta, theologian, makes the following observation concerning the origins of human life in water: "All life is pregnant in intimacy... Everything that is, began in intimacy. We swim in the cosmic amniotic fluid; we are connected through an umbilicus to the Nameless who is intimacy itself."[14]

Sound travels four times faster in water than in air. The vibratory Qi engendered by tuning forks, due to its capacity to reach every cell via specialized conduits of water, penetrates the deepest recesses of the body, thus making tuning forks ideal for use in transformative protocols.

The Kidneys store essence and connect to the bone and bone marrow. Our skeletal structure can be viewed as a dynamic sound conduction system within the body, transporting healing vibrations throughout it with remarkable efficiency. In its functioning as an organic sounding board, bone directly impacts the Kidney meridian and the Water element.

A balanced Water person has determination, willpower, resourcefulness, stamina, ingenuity, adaptability, and the capacity to easily embrace change. When imbalanced, they are insecure, lethargic, fearful, phobic, overwhelmed, depressed, and rigid. The wisdom of the Water element reminds us to rest, balance, and conserve Kidney Qi and essence during the winter months to recharge our Zhi.

Water Element Imbalances

An imbalance of the Water element is indicated in issues such as osteoarthritis, osteoporosis, adrenal insufficiency, and organic hormonal imbalances, as well as similar imbalances resulting from the abuse of synthetic steroids, addictions to opiates such as morphine, codeine, and heroin, and pain-relieving analgesic medications like fentanyl and other opioids. Symptoms may include lower back pain, muscle aches due to calcium deficiency, arthritic knee joints, and neck pain.

Patients who exhibit low energy will often ingest stimulants, like caffeine, from coffee and other sources, so as to maintain a level of maximum alertness and responsiveness. Kidney imbalances develop from shock, stress, and trauma experienced over a long period of time; this gives rise to adrenal insufficiency.

Japanese Water Element Hara Palpation

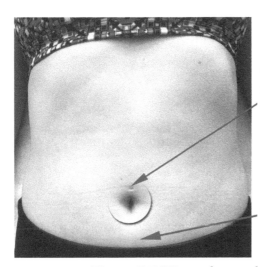

Tightness around the umbilicus, Kid-16 Huangshu or Kid-15½, Zhongzhu

Weak, cottony Dantien

Figure 7.7 *Water element hara*

Location: Palpate Kid-16 Huangshu, Vitals Shu 0.5 cun on both sides of the navel for tightness, tenderness, or a lumpy sensation. Then palpate Kid-15½ Zhongzhu, Middle Flow 1.5 cun below Kid-16 Huangshu, bilaterally, for tenderness and/or emptiness, which can indicate adrenal deficiency. When palpating under the navel, you may find a weak, cottony sensation.

If this area is tight or tender, treat the following.

1. TCM Kid-27 Shufu, Shu Mansion; located 2 cun on either side of the sternum, in the depression on the lower border of the clavicle.

2. TCM Kid-6 Zhaohai, Shining Sea, 1 cun below the prominence of the medial malleolus (internal ankle bone).

Japanese Treatment for Adrenal Insufficiency

This Kidney adrenal treatment addresses:

- adrenal gland exhaustion

- trauma, shock, fright, depression

- severe allergies

- life-threatening experience

- natural hormone production

- lower back pain, infertility, and impotence.

Japanese Treatment Points for Adrenal Exhaustion

TCM Kid-6 Zhaohai, Shining Sea is 1 cun below the prominence of the medial malleolus (internal ankle bone).

TCM Kid-27 Shufu, Shu Mansion is under the clavicle 2 cun on either side of the sternum (breastbone), on the lower border of the clavicle.

Needling technique: Bilaterally needle TCM Kid-6 Zhaohai, angling the needle up toward the head. Bilaterally needle TCM Kid-27 Shufu horizontally toward the sternum and the Ren Mai meridian. When a patient has adrenal deficiency, it is best to support and consolidate essence, rather than to disperse it by needling outward from the sternum.

Tuning forks: Vibrate the Acutonics Ohm® Unison tuning forks, one on TCM Kid-6 Zhaohai in the ankle, and the other on TCM Kid-27 Shufu under the clavicle. Treat bilaterally. Resonate the tuning forks on the indicated points three times.

Tuning forks and acupuncture needles: Needle the point first, then resonate the tuning fork around the needle for patients who are severely adrenal deficient. Do not combine these modalities until you have treated the patient several times; it may be too exhausting for them.

Conclusion

This chapter is unique in that it provides you, the reader, with a variety of protocols based upon Five Element theory, drawing upon its traditional elemental correspondences and coupling these theoretical considerations with practical Japanese treatments based upon hara palpation. You have a choice of using tuning forks or acupuncture needles (if you're an acupuncturist), or combining the two modalities.

Vibrational hara encourages the development of receptivity, the art of listening, in the practitioner, so that you may become as attuned to elemental imbalances as the blind *ammas* in Japan are when palpating the abdomens of *their* patients. This skill set facilitates the heightening of intuitive awareness and fosters dedication to a conscious practice of being present and grounded within one's body.

Perhaps, at this point, you may share some of the disorientation that I experienced in attempting to navigate those narrow streets of Tokyo back in the 1980s, when my Western linear mind was short-circuited by an absence of verbal information, and I was compelled to resort to a more instinctual means of moving through my environment.

My studies of Japanese acupuncture with such noted senseis as Kiiko Matsumoto and Shudo Denmei, and an earlier immersion in Zen shiatsu with Shizuto Masunaga and Wataru Ohashi, have done much to facilitate the continuing reprogramming of my consciousness. I have realized that touch, awareness, and receptivity are essential to the healing process. I encourage you to be open to this idea, this alternative paradigm of engagement with your patients, to allow yourselves to "get lost," become confused, and forge a new path of healing that embraces a nonviolent way of being present in the world.

Chapter 8

Solo Sound Therapy Treatments

Tell me, I'll forget,
Show me, I will remember;
but involve me, and I'll understand.

Chinese proverb

This chapter is written with an "ear" to the treatment of "super-sensitive," "needle-phobic" patients, and also for non-acupuncturists who may wish to take advantage of these non-needle protocols. All of the acu-sound treatments in this book can be integrated into an acupuncture, massage, physiotherapy, chiropractic, music therapy, or psychotherapeutic practice.

Self-Medication

These tuning fork protocols are perfect for self-treatment, especially the Grounding Protocol: A Vibratory Ritual of Earthing. For example, after a long flight, when the body's biorhythms are out of sync, self-treatment with the Acutonics Ohm® Unison tuning fork combination resonating on the points provided for the Grounding Protocol can assist with the restoration of balance and harmony.

There are three sound protocols that will be highlighted in this chapter. *We recommend that you perform these treatments with tuning forks only.*

- The Grounding Protocol: A Vibratory Ritual of Earthing: This treatment is incorporated at the beginning and end of each session. The Acutonics Ohm® Unison and the Acutonics® Low Ohm Unison tuning fork sets are resonated upon the indicated acupuncture points and chakric energy centers. The seven primary chakras are the principal loci of the human energy field, which emanate from distinct anatomical areas that are usually depicted on the ventral side of the body. They range along the midline from the top of the head to the soles of the feet.

◈ The Sacred Mudra Ritual: Lacing the Three Jiaos: This ritual combines Taoist alchemical practices with Hindu sacred hand positions, otherwise known as mudras. This treatment is only effective in tuning fork applications, due to their vibratory nature.

◈ The Corpus Callosum: Vibrational Balancing of the Twin Hemispheres of the Brain: This unique ritual will permit you to balance the right, intuitive, and the left, logical, hemispheres of the brain. It is particularly effective in addressing conditions such as dyslexia and other learning disabilities.

In all of these treatments, the indicated acu-sound points overlap with the chakric centers. As is the case with the acupuncture points and meridians, the Hindu chakra system is thousands of years old and, in fact, it predates Chinese medicine. Chakra means "wheel," or "vortex of energy." Each primary chakra corresponds to a location on the spinal column, a nerve plexus, and an endocrine gland. The chakras encode very specific aspects of human psychology and relate to particular life issues and stages of spiritual development. Each chakra has a characteristic color and vibration. Traditionally, the seven chakras represent a microcosm, in that each corresponds to one of the seven planets—Sun, Moon, Mercury, Venus, Mars, Jupiter, Saturn—that were recognized in ancient India, as in the West.

The Grounding Protocol: A Vibratory Ritual of Earthing

Focus upon earthing/grounding your patient prior to beginning the treatment, so that the Yang Qi is rooted and will not rise to the head. If you do not do so, this may contribute to a headache, elevate blood pressure, or trigger hot flashes or the recurrence of psychospiritual issues.

The Acutonics Ohm® Unison tuning forks are resonated three times on each of the energy centers, connecting acupuncture points and chakras simultaneously. This fosters balance in all the chakras. The heart is the bridge between the lower and upper chakras, hence each point combination features Ren-17 Shanzhong, Chest Center. The crown chakra, Du-20 Baihui, Hundred Meetings, is then combined with Ren-17 Shanzhong, and the same procedure is followed with the other chakras.

Table 8.1 The crown chakra: Du-20, Baihui, Hundred Meetings

Location	The vertex (top) of the head on the midline, in the depression 5 cun posterior to the anterior hairline.
[AQ]Crown chakra (Hindu name)	Sahsrara
Color	White/clear
Endocrine gland	Pituitary
Goals	Universal connection

Table 8.2 The heart chakra: Ren-17 Shanzhong, Chest Center

Location	On the midline of the chest, in a depression between the breasts, and level with the fourth intercostal space.
Heart chakra (Hindu name)	Anahata
Color	Green/pink
Endocrine gland	Thymus
Goals	Compassion, forgiveness, relinquishment of the past

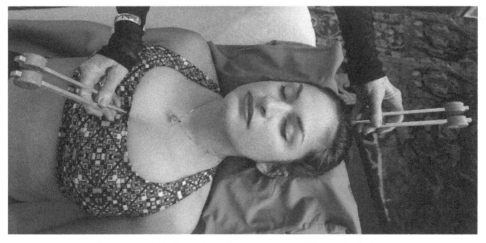

Figure 8.1 *Balancing the crown and heart chakras*

Crown and Heart Chakra: Treatment Protocol

Du-20 Baihui, a point we can associate with the crown chakra, is always resonated upon simultaneously three times with Ren-17 Shanzhong, Chest Center, for the heart chakra. Connecting these two chakras facilitates a dynamic linkage between the head (thinking) and the heart (feeling and compassion). Many people in our culture do not embrace, or connect, their compassionate wisdom with their thinking processes and operate solely from intellectual concerns. They obsess constantly and do not breathe properly. For all intents and purposes, they are nothing more than "floating" heads. This state of affairs has only been exacerbated by the worldwide epidemic of addiction to visual technologies.

The proper inhalation and exhalation of breath grounds the individual in the present moment, and the failure to do so imprisons people within their own minds and detaches them from any vital connection with physical reality. They may feel that they are inhabiting their bodies, and many of them spend thousands of dollars a year perfecting their outer appearance, but the truth of the matter is starkly different. We have encountered individuals who are simply incapable of taking a deep breath in the lower Dantien, i.e., what we as singers would describe as intercostal breathing. While they exhibit wonderfully toned and aesthetically pleasing abdomens, the tonicity of the area is only superficial. The viscera, the organs themselves, starved of vital oxygen, are impaired in their functioning. Consequently, these individuals frequently manifest digestive issues, problems with fertility, etc. Administering this Grounding Protocol as part of your treatment will initiate a process whereby they may begin to reestablish a connection to their vital Qi, prana, pneuma, and Earth, *terra firma*.

The next step in the protocol connects the point for the third eye chakra, Yintang, M-HN-3, Hall of Impression, with Ren-17 Shanzhong.

Table 8.3 The third eye chakra, Yintang, M-HN-3, Hall of Impression

Location	In the glabellar crease at the midpoint of the medial extremities of the eyebrows; calms the Shen, treats insomnia, stress, and melancholy.
Third eye chakra (Hindu name)	Ajna center
Color	Purple
Endocrine gland	Pineal
Goals	Inner vision, integration; when the heart and third eye are connected, it encourages a way of seeing that is nonjudgmental, that partakes of visionary, inspirational, and uplifting qualities

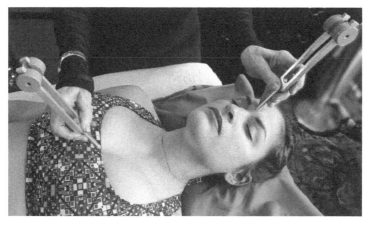

Figure 8.2 *Connecting the third eye with the heart chakra*

Third Eye Chakra: Treatment Protocol

Vibrate the Acutonics Ohm® Unison tuning forks on the third eye and the heart chakra three times simultaneously. Please be mindful of how long the vibration lasts on each point, in other words, how readily your patient is absorbing the frequencies. If the heart center, for example, stops resonating prior to the third eye, then re-apply the tuning fork combination until the resonance "holds," or when you feel that the patient is no longer taking in the vibrations.

Table 8.4 The throat chakra, Ren-22 Tiantu, Heavenly Prominence

Location	The throat area, in the center of the suprasternal fossa.
Throat chakra (Hindu name)	Visuddha
Color	Blue
Endocrine gland	Thyroid
Goals	Creativity, speaking the truth

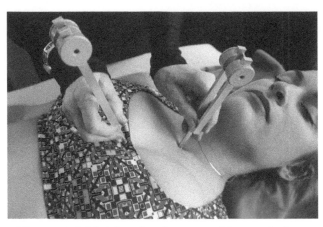

Figure 8.3 *Uniting the throat and heart chakras*

Throat Chakra: Treatment Protocol

The throat chakra, Ren-22 Tiantu, is activated simultaneously with the heart, Ren-17 Shanzhong, Chest Center, so that the patient can give voice to their authentic truth and power. Ren-22 Tiantu is a Windows of the Sky point, which, if imbalanced, results in difficulty expressing oneself and possible depression.

Historically, the throat chakra is a place of blockage, especially for women and the elderly. Their voices are not usually encouraged, nor acknowledged by society. They are regarded as vulnerable and, therefore, not to be respected. Many judgments and projections are lodged in the throat. Children are "labeled," i.e., classified as the "smart" one, the "creative" child, or, in a reprehensible manner, the "slow" one who will never succeed. This naming wounds the soul and becomes a toxic code that invades the cells, initiating a negative programming that disrupts the DNA.

Many women are afraid to speak their truth for fear of censure, and most of them do not even know how their voices truly sound. They parrot the repetitive and self-sabotaging mantras, such as "I'm sorry... it's my fault," which they have absorbed from their parents, partners, or colleagues. Women and men who are unconventional, pursue alternative gender choices, or who are gentle and creative are often shunned or simply denied the opportunities to express themselves in the world.

The elderly, who are closer to death, can be a source of discomfort to people who worship at the fountain of youth and so-called "beauty." These individuals are terrified of the implications of death—release, surrender, and gentle acceptance—and, in their fear, they lose the capacity to claim, and share, the personal wisdom that may be acquired as part of the organic process of maturation. They avoid the elderly and less fortunate as they would a virulent disease, suppressing in their conscious awareness the ultimate and inescapable truth: we all die. Every organic life-form on this planet is subject to the dictates of mortality, and it is a measure of the pathology of our youth-obsessed culture that there are those individuals who refuse to surrender to the rhythms of the natural order.

The ancient Chinese, from their observations of nature over the centuries, understood the changing of the seasons and incorporated this consideration into their Five Element theory, which we discussed in Chapter 7. They honored the progression from spring to winter, birth to old age, and knew that, at the end of the journey, it was time to go within, reap the harvest of wisdom gained from experience, and claim their spiritual maturity.

Wounding to the throat chakra, which we have encountered time and again with students in our seminars, is perhaps the most debilitating of all psychospiritual burdens. The throat is the conduit for our emerging sense of self, the means whereby we stake our individual claim upon physical reality. The capacity to give voice to our yearnings, to communicate the outpourings of our inner creative being, whether it be through words, music, new ideas and concepts, or inventions, often cannot withstand the damage that has been done by those who, by rights, should have been our most stalwart defenders. The voice, in the same manner as our face, is one of the most personal aspects of who we are; the pain that results from its being suppressed, silenced, ridiculed, or ignored invariably haunts the unfortunate souls who have endured these traumas throughout their lives.

It may be instructive to share a compelling example: we had occasion to work with a practitioner who was from a family of singers. The father, a professional singer himself, had taken elaborate pains to prohibit his children from pursuing that same career path. One of the symptoms of a blocked throat chakra is the appearance of a double chin, which may have nothing to do with actual accumulation of weight but, in fact, is the result of preverbal tension[1] or other injury to the throat chakra. This was largely the case with our student; the suppression of her voice by her father had stymied her personal self-expression.

We treated her with tuning forks, using a unique technique we refer to as Vibrational Somato-Emotional Release, or VSER. The blockages under the chin were resonated upon, while she simultaneously made nonverbal sounds. In that moment, a voice of authentically Wagnerian proportions emerged from her throat with consummate ease. It was astonishing, and we were genuinely grieved that such a magnificent natural instrument would have been denied the opportunity to be developed to its fullest extent. The energetic opening that she experienced in the seminar proved to be authentically transformative, and the impact upon other aspects of her life was extraordinary. When we next saw her, we were greeted by a poised, glamorous, beautiful woman who had, as she put it, been reborn. The treatment had served as a powerful catalyst for a dynamic process of self-reclamation.

Sacral (Sexual) Chakra: Treatment Protocol

The next step of the protocol is to establish a link between the Heart, Ren-17 Shanzhong, Chest Center, and Ren-4 Guanyuan, Gate of Origin.

Table 8.5 The sacral (sexual) chakra, Ren-4 Guanyuan, Gate of Origin

Location	3 cun below the navel; this point tonifies original Qi, benefits essence and nourishes the Kidneys and the Uterus. It roots the ethereal soul, which does not die, according to Chinese Taoist philosophy.
Sacral (sexual) chakra (Hindu name)	Svadhisthana
Color	Orange
Endocrine gland	Gonads, ovaries
Goals	Sensuality, pleasure, reproduction

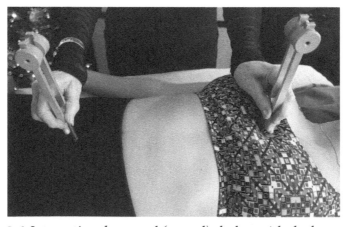

Figure 8.4 *Integrating the sacral (sexual) chakra with the heart chakra*

In describing the psychospiritual attributes of the Ren Mai in Chapter 3, we alluded to the "creative/procreative duality." This energetic resonance between the throat chakra and the sexual chakra encodes a potential conflict between the instinctual urge to reproduce and the expression of an individualized creativity that is independent of the dictates of evolution.

In midlife, after having fulfilled their biological responsibility as mothers to the next generation, women often develop blockages within the throat chakra. These may be due to societal pressures or simply their own intuitive and protective reaction to untold millennia of suppression of the feminine voice. These disharmonies often manifest as hormonal imbalances that affect the metabolism of the thyroid gland and energetic conditions that compromise the throat. Ultimately, these can be seen as the result of a not-so-subtle disempowerment and the reluctance to transgress social and familial boundaries for fear of censure.

In this context, it is interesting to add that our throat-chakra-blocked patient, subsequent to her treatment with us, reported a similar opening of the sexual chakra a few months later when, after this energetic shift, she had occasion to sing for her partner, who said that he "heard" her voice for the first time! Such a phenomenon further illustrates the vital linkage between the two chakras, and the fact that a blocked throat chakra can deprive the individual of a voice to which others pay heed.

Table 8.6 Root chakra, Kid-1 Yongquan, Gushing Spring

Location	On the soles of the feet, between the second and third metatarsal bones. It calms the spirit and revives consciousness. This point represents pure, natural water, life force, power, rebirth, and regeneration. It clears the brain; if there is too much energy in the head at Du-20 Baihui, Kid-1 Yongquan will descend the Qi and ground the person involved.
Root chakra (Hindu name)	Muladhara
Color	Red
Endocrine gland	Adrenals
Goals	Life force, grounding, attending to basic needs

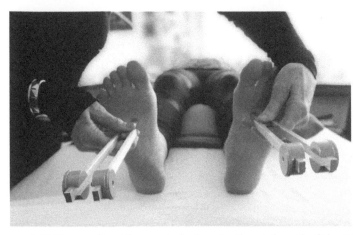

Figure 8.5 *Grounding the root chakra in the rich soil of the Earth*

The Sacred Mudra Ritual: Lacing the Three Jiaos ————

This innovative treatment involves a process of interlacing the three San Jiaos or Three Heaters of Chinese medicine, using tuning forks to activate the relevant treatment points. The treatment is enhanced with Hindu sacred mudra hand positions that are formed by the patient. According to Gertrud Hirschi, mudras "signify a gesture, a mystic position of the hands, a seal, body postures and breathing techniques... Specific positions can lead to the states of consciousness that they symbolize."[2]

She cites an example of a person who wishes to be freed of fear, and in passionately practicing the mudra for fearlessness, she will be, in time, released from this negative emotion. In India, mudras are a recognized aspect of religious ceremonies, and they depict the Hindu gods via their specific hand postures. Mudras are used in Indian dance movements and integrated in the practice of tantric yoga. They also are an important component of Buddhist spiritual observances.

The other component of this unusual vibrational treatment, activation of the San Jiao and the Three Heaters of the body, is drawn from Taoist philosophy and Chinese medicine. "The translation of the ideogram representing the San Jiao is the 'three burners' or 'three cauldrons,' the three 'combustion ovens.'"[3]

In Taoism, the three heaters are actively involved in the alchemical transformation of body/mind/spirit. The proto-scientific pursuit of alchemy is one of the more profound legacies of the ancient world, one that encompasses several philosophical traditions spanning some four millennia and three continents. One suggested stream of etymology of the modern English word *alchemy* pinpoints its origins in ancient Egypt, from the Arabic word *al-kimia*, derived from *al-Khem*. Contact between China and the Arabic world may have resulted in the transmission of alchemical writings to the East; in the early Tang Dynasty (8th century CE), the word *kiem-yak* was used to describe the "golden elixir" that was the essence of immortality.

Khem was the ancient Arabic word for Egypt, which may have originally referred to the rich, black soil of the Nile Delta, the fertile muck from which sprang the entirety of Egyptian civilization. The annual rebirth of life from this primeval ooze, flooded by the abundant waters of the Nile at the time of the heliacal rising of the star Sirius, provides us with a central image of, and philosophical motivation for, the alchemical art; that of the resurrection of both body and spirit.

Like Western alchemists, the earliest Chinese practitioners of the art sought to liberate spirit from matter by subjecting it to a variety of chemical processes. This included heating lead or a similar unrefined substance, the *prima materia*, in a large sealed furnace, or retort, so as to burn off the dross and ultimately transform that raw material into gold.

They later evolved in their understanding of the practice to embrace the idea that they could perform similar operations of transformation upon themselves within the body; the alchemical "fire" embodied in three *internal* anatomical burners would permit them to achieve immortality, a spiritual "gold" that was incorruptible and undying.

The ancient Chinese believed that the desired goal of alchemy, as they saw it, immortality, could be achieved through actual physical transformation. The alchemical vessel, the cauldron or retort, became the three heaters, situated in the lower, middle, and upper area of the body's torso.

In the Han Dynasty (3rd century BCE), Wai-dan, or external alchemy, encouraged the consumption of toxic materials—mercury, in the form of cinnabar—to provoke the alchemical fire for the purpose of transforming Shen, spirit.

Later in the Sung Dynasty (11th century CE), Nei-dan, or inner alchemy, was developed. These later practitioners recognized that it was no longer necessary to effect alchemical change internally through the transformation of external substances; they advocated, instead, the use of more practical tools, such as visualization, breathing techniques, meditation, acupuncture, herbs, and, most important, interlacing the three Jiaos, starting in the lower heater. The goal was a return to a primordial state, "the face before they were born," and to embody spirit in physical form.

Lower Heater

The lower heater is in the lower abdomen and relates to the functions of the Kidneys, Intestines, and reproductive organs. The treatment point is Ren-4 Guanyuan, Gate of Origin, which is on the midline, 3 cun below the navel. This is the Dantien, the source of original Qi, the Front Mingmen, and the mu of the Small Intestine meridian: "'Mu' means to gather or to collect, and the Front mu points are where the Qi of the zangfu [Yin and Yang organs] gathers on the anterior surface of the body."[4]

This important point is also designated as the Cinnabar Field, and Sea of Blood, because it relates to the Uterus and reproduction. The name of the point further illustrates its association with alchemical practice. Cinnabar is a compound of mercury, mercury sulphide, with a lustrous bright red color, hence the symbolic linkage with menstrual blood. In Western alchemy, mercury, in the form of the god Hermes Trismegistus (Thrice-Great Hermes), had dominion over the alchemical processes, and the element of mercury itself, quicksilver, was considered one of the three indispensable alchemical substances, with sulfur and salt. Alchemists regarded mercury as the *prima materia* from which all metals were formed. They believed that different metals could be produced by varying the quality and quantity of sulfur contained within the mercury.

Many alchemists would similarly ingest mercury as part of their own process of inner transformation and, regrettably, poisoned themselves with the metal, which is highly toxic. The external use of cinnabar still occurs in various feng shui rituals in China and elsewhere. In Qi-gong and Tai Chi, the Dantien is the center of life force and breath, and serves as a grounding point for Qi. This source of original Qi benefits essence, nourishes Kidney Yin and strengthens Kidney Yang, calms the Shen, and roots the ethereal soul, which relates to the Hun, the soul that does not die.

The Pyramid Position

The mudra hand position for the lower heater forms an inverted triangle. To create this configuration, the two thumbs are aligned directly under the navel, with their tips touching, while the remaining fingers point downward toward the pubic bone.

The Acutonics Ohm® Unison tuning fork combination is vibrated three times in the center of the triangle on the point Ren-4 Guanyuan. The downward-pointing figure is a symbol of the Fire element, the color red, and blood, reminding us that this is the Cinnabar Field, Blood Chamber, and the Uterus, the seat of new life. It also signifies the process of reproduction in both sexes.

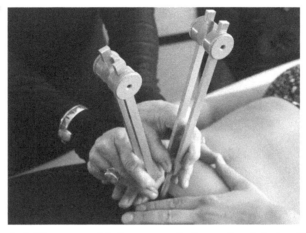

Figure 8.6 *The pyramid shape reminds us that Mother Earth is the creatrix and her womb holds the seed for all new life*

Middle Heater

The middle heater is found on the upper level of the abdomen, and it represents the functioning of the Spleen and Stomach. The treatment points are TH-2 Yemen, Fluid Gate; they are located between the ring and little finger on both hands, 0.5 cun proximal to the margin of the web.

TH-2 Yemen is a Ying Spring point, which clears heat in the body, and also the Water point of the Fire channel, which transports fluids upward to the face and head. This action cools and calms patients who exhibit red faces and dry eyes, who are agitated, nervous, frightened, and Shen-disturbed.

Psychospiritual applications of TH-2 Yemen include the treatment of patients who cannot "go with the flow"—who lack fluidity in their lives. The use of tuning forks, rather than needles, further instills the qualities of the Water element to cool and tranquilize these patients.

The Prayer Position

The mudra hand posture for the middle heater is the prayer position, which evokes qualities of respect, humility, and surrender to the Divine Source. Both hands are placed in prayer position over the solar plexus, at Ren-12 Zhongquan, Middle Cavity. It is located on the midline, 4 cun above the navel.

While the patient's hands are in prayer position, one of the two Acutonics Ohm® forks is placed upon TH-2 Yemen, on the one hand, and the other fork on the same point on the opposite hand. The patient will feel the vibration passing through the hands, especially in the chakras located in the palms. Treat this point combination three times to achieve the desired result. This mudra position facilitates an attitude of humility and respect, allowing a new consciousness to emerge.

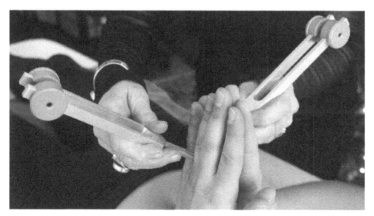

Figure 8.7 *The Prayer Position reminds us to surrender*

The Upper Heater

The upper heater is located in the upper thorax, where the heart and lung organs reside. The targeted area for the treatment is Ren-17 Shanzhong, the Front Mu of the Pericardium, which wraps around and protects the Heart. Once again, it is located in the depression between the breasts, at the level of the fourth intercostal space.

Ren-17 Shanzhong is a key acu-sound point in the Grounding Protocol, and it continues to be an important treatment location in this final component of the Sacred Mudra Ritual.

The Pericardium cushions the Heart against the emotional blows and difficulties encountered in life. It is therefore referred to as the Heart Protector, and it also regulates and gathers Qi in the chest, aiding in maximal efficiency of breathing, i.e., breathing freely and fully.

The Inner Child Position

This final mudra hand position engages the inner child and evokes a state of innocence and qualities of truth and unconditional love for the self and others. It protects the heart chakra, encouraging the release of old wounds and resentments.

Both hands, palm side down, are crossed over the chest, in the Ren-17 Shanzhong area. The two Acutonics Ohm® forks are then resonated upon the paired SI-6 Yanglao, Support the Aged, points, three times bilaterally. SI-6 Yanglao is located in the hollow on the radial side of the styloid process of the ulna.

This point encourages a process of healthy aging and aids people with vision problems, muscle and joint pain, skin rashes, liver spots (hyperpigmentation), sleep issues, and general dryness. It is regarded as a longevity point, the treatment of which helps anyone, regardless of their age, to feel and look healthy. It also fosters a vital connection to their inner, original child, who is creative, alive, and vibrant.

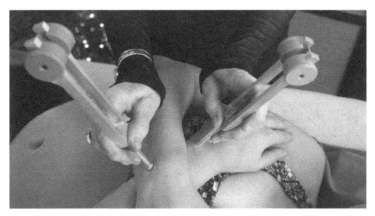

Figure 8.8 *The Inner Child Position supports ageless aging and creativity*

The three different heaters work together in intertwined and unified function. The lower heater is operative in the functioning of the middle heater, which, in turn, acts upon the upper heater, which influences the lower heater. The result of this multiple dovetailing is an intermixing of all bodily energies moving toward the precise goals of each organ's special utilization.

> By virtue of its central function, the triple heater is like an orchestra conductor, articulating the gifts of the hereditary energies in the outcome of the acquired energies (those from food and respiration).[5]

The final solo sound treatment that we are offering to you in this chapter involves balancing the twin hemispheres of the brain via the corpus callosum.

Corpus Callosum Vibrational Balancing Treatment ———

The corpus callosum plays an important role in balancing the two cerebral hemispheres of the brain. It is the largest commissure of the cortex, and the commissure fibers crossing through the corpus callosum connect the cortices of both hemispheres.

The right brain relates to our intuitive, creative, emotional, and nonlinear brain. It develops prior to birth and plays a significant role *in utero* and in early childhood. It is particularly relevant to:

- the perception of shapes and eye/hand coordination

- emotional development

- sensitivity to emotions expressed by the voice (especially that of the mother) and by music

- bodily sensations and feeling awareness.

In contrast, the left brain is logical, factual, intellectual, rational, verbal, and linear. We might categorize the right brain as more Yin and receptive, and the left as Yang and active. Neuroscientist Antonio Damasio demonstrated that anyone who has developed a cerebral lesion following a stroke or accident and has lost physical sensation will exhibit a parallel loss of emotional expression. The body houses the emotions, either directly, or through their representations of the somato-sensational structures of the brain.[6]

We have observed that, historically, women have been called upon to multitask more than men. They have used their intuitive, emotional brains to nurture and support their children and their logical, linear brains to make important practical decisions for their families.

Of course, this situation is changing with contemporary men sometimes functioning as stay-at-home dads, who may previously have been employed in corporate environments or who still maintain such employment. We should also point out that individuals who routinely exercise their right-brain functions, be they men or women, such as musicians, artists, or intuitive consultants, may also exhibit more balance between the two hemispheres. In his book *Musicophilia*, the late neurologist and writer Oliver Sacks reports a study published in 1995 by researcher Gottfried Schlaug, of Harvard University, that demonstrates that various structures of the brain, including the corpus callosum, are visibly enlarged in the brains of professional musicians.[7]

In our *Facial Soundscapes*™ seminars we routinely instruct our students in the rudiments of physiognomy, and the difference in functioning between the two halves of the face. The right side of the face is linked to the left brain, and the left side to the right brain. This asymmetry in terms of neural connection is directly related to the qualities of the disparate hemispheres.

The right side of the face, due to its connection with the linear left brain, is more concerned with perception by others: "How do I wish the world to see me, and what do I want to project to the outside world?" Hence, it is what we would describe as the public side of the face. It is perhaps not surprising that this is usually the face that we show to the camera or the audience if we are in the business of portraying ourselves to others. Every actor has a "good" side, which is usually the right side.

Conversely, the left side of the face, linked to the right brain, relates more to our sense of ourselves when we are alone. The disparities between the two sides of the face can be quite revealing, because they illustrate potential conflicts between public perception and comfort with the role we play in society, and the quality of our private lives.

Corpus Callosum Balancing Treatment

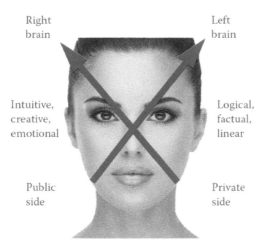

Figure 8.9 *The Corpus Callosum Balancing treatment balances the intuitive and logical hemispheres of the brain*

In addressing this question of right/left imbalance, we utilize a special corpus callosum point, which is located along the length of the tragus cartilage in front of the ear. It affects the laterality of the two cerebral hemispheres.

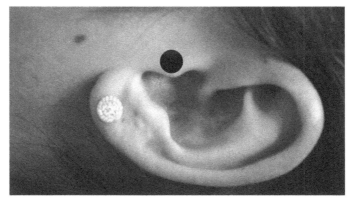

Figure 8.10 *The corpus callosum auricular treatment point*

Once again, we utilize our Acutonics Ohm® Unison tuning fork combination, which is initially employed as a diagnostic tool, to discern which side of the brain needs balancing. This works in two ways: the patient listens to the resonance bilaterally, and the practitioner can sense when the vibration is more readily absorbed by one ear than the other, i.e., if it stops sooner.

Instructions

1. Have the patient listen to the Acutonics Ohm® Unison tuning forks, three times.

2. Note which side absorbs the resonance faster, the right or left ear. For example, if the tone being resonated by the left ear disappears quicker, this is indicative of an imbalance with the right, nonlinear, creative brain. If the converse is true, then the left brain is the one that is in need of attention.

3. For the treatment, place one Ohm fork on Du-20 Baihui, located on the midline at the vertex (top) of the head, in the depression 5 cun posterior to the anterior hairline. The other fork is then vibrated on the corpus callosum point, which is situated in front of the tragus cartilage of the ear. Apply the frequency simultaneously to both points, until the duration of vibration is no longer different, or the sound is no longer being absorbed.

   For example, when the patient is listening, if the vibrations cease sooner on the right side, place one Ohm fork on Du-20 Baihu, Hundred Meetings at the crown of the head and the other on the *right* corpus callosum point in front of the tragus cartilage. Note, however, that you should balance both points. As previously established, the right ear is associated with the left brain, therefore you are addressing an imbalance of that hemisphere.

   It is invariably the case these days that patients who work in corporate environments exhibit fatigue of the left brain, caused by an excess of linear thinking. This treatment will redress this disharmony and permit Qi to flow more readily to both brain hemispheres.

This is a wonderfully effective vibrational treatment that allows you to successfully rebalance your patients' brains, and treat people with more serious syndromes, including learning disorders such as dyslexia and autism. It is an extremely useful and unusual approach, and as effective as it is elegant.

We usually start a treatment session with this Corpus Callosum Balancing treatment, and then follow it with the Grounding Protocol. The Sacred Mudra ritual can then be integrated into the balance of the treatment, should you determine that your patient requires it. Note again that all these protocols are for sound treatment only with Acutonics Ohm® tuning forks. Your patients, or your friends and family, will find them to be quite beneficial. You can also self-medicate with any of them, although you would need help from a colleague for the Sacred Mudra ritual.

Remember that you are in little danger of overtreating with these vibrational protocols, due to the adaptogenic nature of sound vibration, so you may treat yourself and your patients without undue concern.

As the practitioner, we remind you to be receptive, aware, and, most important, breathe into your Dantien, so that you will be thoroughly grounded and thus able to function as an effective transmitter of the healing vibrations.

Summary of Treatment Procedures
The Grounding Protocol: A Vibratory Ritual of Earthing
Instructions: Vibrate the Acutonics Ohm® Unison tuning forks loose simultaneously three times on the pairs of points in Table 8.7.

Table 8.7 Points for the Grounding Protocol

Crown chakra	Du-20 Baihui, Hundred Meetings	and	Ren-17 Shanzhong, Chest Center	Heart chakra
Third eye chakra	Yintang, M-HN-3, Hall of Impression	and	Ren-17 Shanzhong, Chest Center	Heart chakra
Throat chakra	Ren-22 Tiantu, Heavenly Prominence	and	Ren-17 Shanzhong, Chest Center	Heart chakra
Sexual chakra	Ren-4 Guanyuan, Gate of Origin	and	Ren-17 Shanzhong, Chest Center	Heart chakra
Root chakra	Kid-1 Yongquan, Gushing Spring		Vibrate the Acutonics® Low Ohm tuning forks bilaterally, one on the sole of each foot	

The Sacred Mudra Ritual: Lacing the Three Jiaos

Instructions: Vibrate the Acutonics Ohm® Unison tuning forks simultaneously three times on the indicated points; start with the lower heater and work upward.

Table 8.8 Points for the Sacred Mudra Ritual

Upper Heater: The Inner Child Position	Ren-17 Shanzhong, Chest Center
	Mudra posture; hands crossed over the chest/heart area
	Treatment points: SI-6 Yanglao, Support the Aged
	The original inner child
Middle Heater: The Prayer Position	Ren-12 Zhongquan, Middle Cavity
	Mudra posture: prayer position
	Treatment points: TH-2 Yemen, Fluid Gate
	Respect, humility, and prayer
Lower Heater: The Pyramid Position	Ren-4 Guanyuan, Gate of Origin
	Mudra posture: an inverted pyramid (triangle)
	Treatment point: Ren-4 Guanyuan, Gate of Origin
	Passageway of original Qi, the Blood Chamber, immortal embryo, breath, and the Dantien

Chapter 9

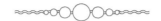

Vibrational Topical and
Internal Treatments

*Don't bend; don't water it down, don't try to make it logical; and
don't edit your soul according to the fashion.*

Franz Kafka

This chapter will introduce both topical and internal protocols using
natural, organic vibrational products to enhance the efficacy of your
treatments, for both you and your patients. You can also synergize the
use of Acutonics® tuning forks and/or acupuncture needling with these
remedies.

We will be discussing the following vibrational remedies:

⬦ the QuintEssentials™ 5 Element Planetary Gem Elixirs

⬦ VibRadiance™ 5 Element Planetary Essential Oils 2 oz bottles and
⅓ oz roller bottles, infused with gem essence

⬦ organic Bulgarian rose moisturizing crème, *Crème Vitale ESP
Rose*

⬦ three organic essential oil hydrosols (Bulgarian rose, neroli,
lavender).

The QuintEssentials™ 5 Element Planetary Gem Elixirs –
These gem elixirs are unique vibrational formulations, whose significance derives from Five Element theory and associated planetary
correspondences that originally appeared in the classic Chinese medicine

text, the *Nei Jing*. As is consistent with Chinese medicine theory, which is organized largely around pentads (aggregates of five), the Chinese chose to consign the Sun and Moon, the Lights of the Heavens, to the recognizable polarities of Yang and Yin. The Sun became the TaiYang (Great Yang) and the Moon the Taiyin (Great Yin). The remaining five visible planets were then associated with the Five Elements, as follows:

- Mercury: Water

- Venus: Metal

- Mars: Fire

- Jupiter: Wood

- Saturn: Earth.

The Latin phrase *quinta essentia* means "fifth element," and the modern English word *quintessence*, from which it derives, has evolved to mean the fundamental nature of a thing, its quiddity, or what we might amusingly term its "thing-ness." However, the term was originally employed by medieval alchemists to refer to a similar, or identical, substance believed to comprise the heavenly bodies or the cosmos. They proposed that a minute portion, a scintilla, of the quintessence was present in all living things on Earth, and that terrestrial affairs could be impacted by cosmic effects. This is one of the cornerstones of astrological theory in both East and West. The principal axiom of the *Corpus Hermeticum*, a body of alchemical writings believed to originate with Hermes Trismegistus (Thrice-Great-Hermes), is "As above, so below." This famous utterance suggests that human beings are a reflection in matter of the perfect ethereal realm of the cosmos.

As living embodiments of the universe, human beings express in their anatomy, physiology, and psychology the archetypal attributes and qualities of the heavenly bodies. This understanding is an essential component of Western medical astrology, the traditional medicine of the West, and it is likewise expressed in Chinese medicine's Five Element theory.

Another meaning of *quinta essentia* is crucial to an understanding of alchemical practice in the West and East; it was considered to be synonymous with the *lapis philosophorum*, the philosopher's stone, or the "golden elixir" of Chinese alchemy.

The philosopher's stone is a legendary alchemical substance that purportedly possessed the capacity to transform base metals such as mercury into gold or silver, a process referred to as *chrysopoeia*, which literally means to "make gold." However, the ultimate objective of the alchemical art was not merely the production of gold from worthless matter; the alchemist also embarked upon a spiritual journey in quest of the *lapis*, the elixir of life, the ingestion of which would provoke a miraculous process of cellular regeneration. This would, in effect, guarantee one's immortality. There was no nobler endeavor than to dedicate one's life to the production of this wondrous substance; hence, alchemy itself was known as the *magnum opus*, the "great work."

In Taoist philosophy, the Golden Elixir, or Golden Pill, represents immortality, openness, selflessness, and unified energy. According to Liu-i-ming of the Complete Reality Taoist tradition, "This pill is completely non-existent, yet it contains ultimate being; it is completely empty, yet in contains fulfillment...try to describe it, and you lose it; whatever you say about it, it is not it."[1] Ancients drew it as a circle and gave it the name "Tao," open selflessness, primal unified energy, the infinite, the great ultimate.[2]

Although Western esotericism, including astrology, is generally organized around a tetrad of elements, Plato, in his book *Timaeus*, introduced the idea of a fifth element, ether. Plato's student Aristotle later identified ether with the quintessence. This *quinta essentia* is believed to unite the other four elements, and is sometimes depicted as the focal point of the five, an arrangement that duplicates the original Chinese medicine schema of the Five Elements that placed Earth at the center.

The name QuintEssentials™ was expressly selected to evoke these ancient esoteric correspondences—that of the Chinese Five Elements, but also with the implication that these elixirs are, by nature of their association with certain precious gemstones, distillations of both crystalline and planetary essences.

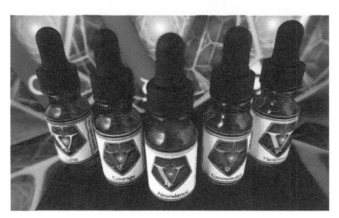

Figure 9.1 *Gem elixirs contain the distilled crystalline essence of a gem or mineral*

What Are Gem Elixirs?

Gem elixirs are vibrational healing remedies that contain the essence of precious gems that have been infused in water and then potentized by the radiance of the Sun and the reflective light of the full Moon. Water is a natural vehicle for the transmission of etheric energies; the process of distillation of the crystalline essence of the gemstone imprints the water with an image of the mineral matrix of its constituents. Each stone possesses distinct healing properties, many of which derive from its frequency, expressed through its apparent color.

Their primary action is to stabilize and balance the energy field; this includes the subtle bodies that comprise the aura and the chakras. They also catalyze and release stress and tension that has accumulated in the energetic structure of the body. As these dissonant energies are discharged, the body's structure realigns itself, and natural balance, stability, and resistance to stress are restored.

It is important to be mindful, when working with gemstones, of the Doctrine of Signatures, i.e., "like attracts like," which stipulates that the various properties of the stone, its color, shape, mineral content, and archetypal qualities correspond with the anatomical component of the body that is affected.

For example, the vibratory remedies of gemstones and sound, produced by a synergy of tuning forks and gems, can be used directly upon the spinal vertebrae to good effect. Bone structure is likewise sensitive to resonance; the back Shu points, which lie along the spinal column, are effective in balancing the function of the internal organs, according to Chinese medicine. A high concentration of neurological tissue in the spinal column can readily transmit healing vibrations to the medulla oblongata, which is important in controlling autonomic nerve function, at one extreme, and the coccyx, at its base.

When gem elixirs are created, the Qi and information from the stones are transferred to the water by a process of distillation. This makes these remedies extremely effective, because both water and gemstones are repositories of memory, transmit intention, and reflect emotions. Homeopathic formulae and flower essences are likewise vibrational healing remedies, but there are distinct differences between them and gem elixirs.

Gem elixirs derive their potency from the crystalline minerals and other matrices of stones, hence their ultimate origin is inorganic, and the properties reflect their birth from the mineral kingdom. In contrast, both homeopathic formulae and flower essences are principally obtained from organic sources.

In our experience, gem elixirs function as a conduit between the organic and inorganic realms of nature, and they have a beneficial impact upon both physical and psychospiritual imbalances. We have witnessed some extraordinary results following the application of gem elixirs upon acu-sound points or when the patient has ingested them internally.

Gem Elixirs in Action

There are two notable instances of cures of acute conditions that we can cite to illustrate the potency of these formulations. The first involves a case of temporary blindness that occurred in a seminar we were teaching in California a few years ago. An acupuncturist, during a group practicum session, was treating wrinkles in the glabellar crease, an area on the face which, from a physiognomical perspective, is associated with the Wood element, and anatomically with the corrugator muscle. In this case, she treated specifically the two parallel lines that can form between the brows, referred to as the "11s."[3] Following the treatment of these lines, the patient reported with some trepidation that she could not see anything; everything was simply a wash of white light. Her ordinary vision was mysteriously obscured.

Although this development was startling, we both intuitively knew that it was an opening of the third eye chakra and heralded a spiritual breakthrough of some significance. It is a truism of metaphysical thought that authentic vision and insight is not a function of the physical eyes. The eyes present us with a distorted view of reality because the images originally transmitted to the brain from the retina via the optic nerve do not reflect what the person ultimately "sees" via the visual processing centers of the cerebral cortex. Our vision is binocular, because the field of vision of the two individual eyes does not coincide, and therefore two different images are presented to the brain for its interpretation. From these conflicting images, it fashions a coherent single representation of the world outside.

Moreover, these overlapping inputs are further divorced from reality because the images that are processed are actually viewed upside down, and then inverted by the brain. Most of us are aware of the phenomenon of optical illusion, which is a result of the idiosyncrasies of our sight. One might argue that, in light of these peculiarities, the visual faculty of human beings, despite our elevation of it to the pinnacle of sensory perception since the time of the Greeks, and ever more so in the modern era, is anything but accurate. It mires our brains in duality, because of the separation of the observer from the observed, and subjects them to misapprehension due to the comparative incoherence of the visual imagery that it perceives.

By way of contrast, it is the pineal gland, our single Cyclopean eye, situated behind the brow at approximately the location of the acupuncture point Yintang, that is the locus of this spiritual vision, a function that we can associate with the third eye, brow, or *ajna* chakra.

We instructed the patients' practitioner to needle GB-37 Guangming, Bright Light, a point on the legs that is an empirical point for the eyes. In addition, we had the patient ingest some of the Jupiter gem elixir, because Jupiter, through its association with Wood, opens to the eyes, and it is also relevant to an expansion of consciousness and both physical and psychospiritual sight.

Upon taking the gem elixir, the patient's vision was immediately restored; even more remarkable, she experienced a considerable heightening of visual acuity, to a degree that she could see easily without her eyeglasses, which she wore at all times. This enhancement of her visual sense was accompanied by an expanded sense of spiritual awareness, a "wide-eyed" openness and altruism, for the first time in her life. She reported seeing auras and was flooded with feelings of optimism and well-being.

The effect persisted for more than a day and, in our estimation, is certainly attributable to the powerful synergy of the gem elixir with the acupuncture needling. The euphoric state of spiritual transcendence that ensued is entirely consistent with the nature of a Jupiterian expansion of consciousness. Thus, the elixir was instrumental in treating the manifest physical symptom, the temporary blindness, as well as the underlying psychospiritual imbalance—lack of faith, suppressed intuition, pessimism, isolation, and rejection.

In another seminar, our assistant of many years, who is usually a tower of strength, was suddenly stricken on the afternoon of the fourth day with uncomfortable sensations of nausea, queasiness, dizziness, cramping, and "clammy" heat. Given the sudden onset of apparent digestive distress, we had her drink some of the Saturn gem elixir in water. We knew that the Saturn elixir would be effective in alleviating these symptoms, because through its Five Element association with Earth, Saturn also relates to the Stomach and Spleen. The instant she drank it, the symptoms vanished.

These immediate cures are exceptional, and they demonstrate the multipronged impact of these powerful vibrational remedies.

Table 9.1 Comparison of vibrational remedies

Homeopathy	Gem elixirs	Flower essences
Organic materials, minerals, herbs (some inorganic) Treats physical and emotional issues	Inorganic material Gemstones Treats physical, emotional, and psychospiritual imbalances More stable than flower essences	Organic material Flowers Treats psychospiritual and emotional issues

Twelfth-century abbess St. Hildegard of Bingen's approach to gem therapy provides us with some of the earliest documented prescriptions of gem waters in the West. Through her experience, she came to recognize that precious stones, being inorganic and thus impervious to decay, distinguish themselves by their stable and balanced nature.

Guidelines for the Use of Gem Elixirs

Vibrational remedies, such as gem elixirs, homeopathy, and flower essences, tend to produce more immediate results than Chinese herbs, which address Qi, blood, fluids, and the realm of the physical body. However, gem elixirs should be ingested or administered more frequently to remain effective.

- Gems should be carefully selected and only those of excellent quality used; none of the gemstones that were chosen for the production of these elixirs are toxic.

- Gems need to be natural, i.e., not irradiated, colored, or treated with wax, resins, or other materials.

- Distilled water ensures the presence of less "programming," or less mineral content, and facilitates the absorption of the gem's information.

- The distilled water containing the gems is then energized in sunlight and later potentized under the light of the full Moon.

- After the gems are removed, the mineral properties and its essence remain imprinted in the water's memory bank.

- Kirlian photography reveals the presence of a ghost-like impression of the stone, accompanied by a trail of light in the water.

- Sometimes a drop of high-quality brandy is added to the gem elixir to preserve its essence and ensure it longevity.

- These gem elixirs are highly concentrated and potent, therefore the dosage, i.e., drops used, is minimal, usually 7 drops under the tongue, three times a day, or mixed in water in a bottle, which may be sipped periodically over the course of the day. They may be taken internally or dropped onto acupuncture or acu-sound points externally.

- These gem elixir formulations last for more than one year.

- They should be stored in a cool, dark place, or in the refrigerator, which will not disturb the integrity of the formulations.

Applications

Gem elixirs can be used internally or externally, mixed with flower essences, homeopathic remedies, or VibRadiance™ 5 Element Planetary Essential Oils for topical application.

Disclaimer: Do not ingest these gem elixirs for the treatment of serious physical ailments, severe mental illness, or during pregnancy. See your medical doctor or health care professional.

EXTERNAL APPLICATIONS

- Use on acupuncture or acu-sound points to enhance the action of these points. Drop the gem elixir on the point first, and then stimulate with acupuncture needles or vibrate with tuning forks.

- Spray them in a room in your home or workplace to clear any negative vibrations.

- Use in a bath (2–4 drops) to revitalize, calm, or lift the spirit.

- Mix them into *Muse L'Herbal USA Crème Vitale ESP Rose* facial moisturizing cream or a body lotion, or add to massage oils to enhance inner and outer beauty.

- Diffuse in the air to uplift the mood, to calm the Shen, and to move, or support, the Qi. Combine the elixir with 2–4 drops of the Muse L'Herbal USA VibRadiance™ 5 Element Planetary Essential Oil of your choice.

Please note: Test for allergic reactions when applying essential oils topically and when spraying or diffusing in the air.

INTERNAL APPLICATIONS

- Use as a therapeutic remedy for physical, emotional, and psychospiritual imbalances.

- Specific gem elixirs can be used as a mouthwash to rinse the teeth, mouth, and gums.

⬧ Add a few drops as an ingredient to enemas to cleanse and detoxify the intestinal tract.

⬧ Use as a douche in the treatment of leukorrhea or vaginitis.

The nature of our formulations and the suggested applications of these gem elixirs are the result of in-depth study of crystals and precious stones, coupled with an understanding of the theory and practice of Chinese medicine, particularly as it pertains to the Five Elements and their planetary correspondences. The traditional correspondences of Western astrological medicine as codified in the doctrine of *melothesia*, in which the signs of the zodiac have anatomical correlates, are similarly relevant to the applications of these planetary formulas. For example, one might utilize the Saturn 5 Element Gem Elixir to address issues that relate to the knees, which are associated with the Western zodiac sign Capricorn, ruled by Saturn, as well as for Earth-element-related imbalances.

In utilizing gem elixirs in your healing practice or for yourself, please be aware that you are employing a dynamic combination of ethereal vibration, planetary archetypes, and mineral intelligence.

Properties and Usage of Gemstones

⬧ Gemstones are an organized principle of life force.

⬧ They act as a portal between the life force of the organic and inorganic realms.

⬧ Gems are inanimate and inorganic, and more stable than the use of flowers, such as orchids.

⬧ The minerals in the gems are amplified and enhance a capacity for awareness rather than bestowing special properties upon people.

We recommend that you cleanse the stones, especially if you live in a highly urbanized environment. In this scenario, the stone may exacerbate the negativity of the environmental toxins. These toxins include air pollution, and especially noise pollution, which is rarely acknowledged but which has profound deleterious impacts upon the health of people subjected to it.

- Cleanse the gems with sea salt, place them in the Sun, or lay them upon an amethyst geode for at least three hours or more.

- The elixirs that we are recommending for your use come in cobalt blue glass bottles with a dropper tip; you can drop a small amount of the appropriate gem elixir on the acu-sound treatment point and then vibrate the Acutonics Ohm® Unison tuning forks three times on that point to balance the organs; you may also treat the Eight Extraordinary meridians to tap into the Jing and the DNA.

- Or, anoint the point with the gem elixir of choice, and needle the point afterwards.

- For a more powerful effect, needle the point, drop the elixir around it, and then resonate the Acutonics Ohm® Unison tuning fork combination on the stem or around the needle.

Gem Elixirs and Chakras

The seven chakras align with acupuncture points along the Ren Mai meridian, on the front of the body. Disharmonies manifesting in these points indicate similar imbalances in the associated chakras. Administering 7 drops of the indicated gem elixir on the chakra, as prescribed below, invariably causes them to realign. The chakra/planet correspondences given below are derived from the Vedic tradition.

- Root chakra: Saturn

- Sexual chakra: Jupiter

- Solar plexus chakra: Mars

- Heart chakra: Venus

- Throat chakra: Mercury

- Third eye chakra: Moon (you could substitute Venus)

- Crown chakra: Sun (you could substitute Jupiter)

Gem elixirs are distilled from gemstones that manifest the colors and properties of the seven principal Hindu chakras.

1. Place the appropriate donut gem on the chakra you wish to treat, and drop the appropriate gem elixir on the acu-sound point.

2. Vibrate the Ohm Unison combination and/or insert needles into the chakra acupuncture point.

Here are some suggested donut gems that may be used on the chakras; we have provided acupuncture points that you may activate via resonance or needling. The placement of these chakric donut gems, for our purposes, is on the ventral side of the body, but they may also be positioned on the back, the dorsal side.

Chakra Donut Gems: Properties

Please note that specific chakra gems have been chosen not only for colors that correspond to those of the chakras, but also by mineral content, archetypal qualities, and historical usage.

Table 9.2 Properties of chakra donut gems

Root/base chakra: Ren-2 Qugu, Curved Bone	**Black onyx** is in the chalcedony quartz family. It centers, grounds, and aligns the individual with higher powers. It helps with self-assertion, boosts confidence and a sense of responsibility, and enhances decision-making, self-control, and good fortune.
Sacral/sexual chakra: Ren-4 Guanyuan, Gate of Origin	**Carnelian** is also a chalcedony (it contains hematite, hence its red color). It: promotes courage, willpower, stability, and sense of community; improves the quality of the blood; stimulates the Small Intestine, metabolism, circulation, and blood flow.
Solar plexus chakra: Ren-12 Zhongquan, Middle Cavity	**Malachite** (alkaline copper carbonate) is a beautiful green stone that can be used to treat the solar plexus and heart chakras. It encourages creativity, leadership, confidence, and emotional clarity; the solar plexus is our power center that psychically protects us, enhancing our willpower, so that we can manifest what we need in the world.
Heart chakra: Ren-17 Shanzhong, Chest Center	**Rose quartz** (pink silicon dioxide) represents compassion, gentleness, and love. It also aids in releasing past wounds.
Throat chakra: Ren-22 Tiantu, Heavenly Prominence	**Lapis lazuli** (lazurite rock; lattice silicate) helps with imbalances related to the throat, larynx, vocal cords, and thyroid glands; it promotes clarity of speech, acceptance, and honesty.
Third eye chakra: Yintang, M-HN-3, Hall of Impression	**Amethyst** (purple silicon dioxide) supports spirituality, meditation, and intuition and aids in releasing addictive emotional patterns.
Crown chakra: Du-20 Baihui, Hundred Meetings	**Clear crystal quartz** (silicon dioxide) is used for spiritual development and to enhance consciousness. It is one of the seven precious stones of Buddhism.

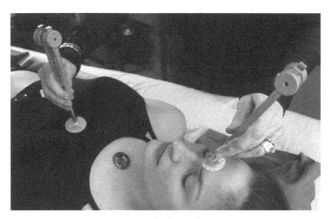

Figure 9.2 *Chakra donut gems*

The QuintEssentials 5 Element Planetary Gem Elixirs Usage and Treatment Protocols

Most of the following gem elixir treatment recommendations have their source in the "natural research" of St. Hildegard of Bingen. In her book *Physica*,[4] she discussed the usage of gemstones to address health imbalances of body and spirit.

St. Hildegard was a woman of the New Age trapped in medieval times. She believed in the interconnectedness of all things in the cosmos, and that, like human beings, the entirety of nature had life force and a soul. She theorized about future "modern" diseases related to loss of spirit, poor diet and nutrition, negative lifestyle choices, stress, and immune system imbalances.

She authored books about cosmic medicine, natural healing, psychotherapy, and healing with gems. According to Dr. Wighard Strehlow, the director of the Hildegard Zentrum Bodensee, in Allensbach, Switzerland, whom we visited on a journey from Zurich to Vienna a few years ago, "Hildegard was one of the first to integrate natural and spiritual healing forces."[5]

We have relied extensively upon Hildegard's pioneering use of this medicine in compiling these treatment recommendations. However, our 5 Element Planetary Gem Elixir remedies also take into consideration Chinese medicine theory, the planetary and zodiacal archetypes of Western astrological medicine, our own study, research, and practical applications of crystals and precious stones in private practice, and experience gained in teaching seminars worldwide.

Some of the gems that Hildegard prescribes in *Physica* for health problems include emerald, onyx, sapphire, topaz, jasper, chalcedony, amethyst, diamond, and quartz crystals. In discussing the beneficial effects of the stone carnelian, she observes that it represents blood: "If blood flows from someone's nose, one should heat wine, place the carnelian in it, and give it to him to drink."[6] As you can observe in Table 9.2, carnelian relates to the sacral/sexual chakra; carnelian contains hematite, a naturally occurring form of iron oxide, which gives the stone a reddish hue and contributes to improved quality of the blood. The acupuncture treatment point recommended is Ren-4 Guanyuan, which is situated in the Dantien, and is also known as Front Mingmen; this area is also referred to as the Cinnabar Field and the Sea of Blood, and it represents the uterus, where life begins.

Another reference that we have found useful is Michael Gienger's *The Healing Crystal First Aid Manual*.[7] Gienger has studied Hildegard's remedies and offers his own twist on how to alleviate the symptoms of various ailments with crystal therapy.

These Five Element planetary remedies can be used to target fundamental disharmonies that may contribute to disease, and they may be employed from either an allopathic or homeopathic perspective. A good example of this would be the treatment of acid reflux or gastroesophageal reflux disease (GERD): the presenting symptom of this digestive syndrome is one of "heat" rising from the stomach through the esophagus into the throat. The allopathic strategy would be to "cool" the heat by means of a cooling planet; in this instance, we would utilize Saturn, because it was originally believed to be cold and dry in nature. Saturn additionally relates to digestion because of the Earth element correlations.

However, in Chinese medicine, the cause of acid reflux is pathogenic heat rising to the Stomach; over time, if unchecked, this heat may damage the Heart. This could contribute to cardiac problems. This phenomenon is referred to as "rebellious Qi." Therefore, the homeopathic approach, "like treating like," would be to reinforce the healthy functioning of the "fire" within the stomach by administering the Mars gem elixir, which relates to the Fire element. In this case, we would recommend using a combination of both elixirs. From the standpoint of Western medical astrology, the blending of Mars/Saturn can be seen to describe the complex of symptoms and underlying constitutional imbalance that contribute to this syndrome.

In the next section, we outline a *materia medica* for our 5 Element Planetary Gem Elixirs that will facilitate effective treatment for the indicated syndromes. We have provided information concerning Five Element and planetary correspondences for each elixir, as each has been distilled from a specific precious stone. Additionally, the section on each gem includes specific correspondences relating to body/mind/spirit.

Note that the recommendations for each syndrome incorporate information from both Five Element theory and Western astrological medicine. Specific dosages for each syndrome are also indicated, i.e., how many drops and how often the elixir should be ingested.

Venus: Metal Element; Diamond

- Mineral: Pure carbon

- Planet: Venus; love, beauty, relationships, compassion vs. narcissism, laziness, lack of depth

GEM: DIAMOND

- Spirit: Compassionate, kind, honest, invincible, spiritual freedom, self-determination, insightful

- Mind: Natural tranquilizer; relieves stress, anxiety, depression

- Body: Strengthens brain, memory, nerves; Treats poor vision, endocrine glands, and blood vessels

SYNDROMES: SPECIFIC RECOMMENDED TREATMENTS

Table 9.3 Arteriosclerosis

Arteriosclerosis	Characterized by cholesterol and calcium deposits in the blood. It decreases circulation to the heart and brain, causing spontaneous thrombosis, heart failure, or an embolism.
Signs and symptoms	Calf pains, cold, bluish limbs, sudden heart pain, decreased physical capacity, poor memory and concentration, dizziness, headache, insomnia, irritability, emotional issues.
Recommendations	Dietary changes: no heavy animal proteins, rather vegetables and foods rich in vitamins C and E; exercise, sleep and rest.
Efficacy of diamond	Breaks down deposits in the blood vessels.

cont.

Dosage	3–7 drops of the gem elixir, three times a day, or work out the daily dosage and add that to water, and sip the liquid all day long.
Hildegard's gem therapy	Place the diamonds in 200–300 ml of water, about 1–1.5 cups, let it set for a day, and drink the diamond water the next day in small sips.

Table 9.4 Gout

Gout	Nitric acid crystals accumulate in the joints, causing inflammation and pain.
Signs and symptoms	Gout deposits are unnoticed until an attack is triggered by an infection, injury, hypothermia, excessive alcohol intake, or acid-forming food.
Recommendations	Dietary changes: a diet with fewer animal proteins, low alcohol intake or none at all; a detoxification diet with plenty of water, rest, and sleep.
Efficacy of diamond	Relieves and treats chronic gout and rheumatic pain.
Dosage	3–7 drops of the gem elixir, three times a day, or work out the daily dosage and add that to water, and sip the liquid all day long.
Hildegard's gem therapy	Place diamonds in 100 ml of water (about 0.5 cup), diluted with white wine, and leave for 24 hours. Drink the diamond water during the following day (while you are making the next batch). Continue this treatment for several months, attend to the dietary and lifestyle changes and emotional imbalances, and all rheumatic symptoms usually vanish. Note: Diamonds bring order and clarity into one's life; they uncompromisingly cleanse what we do not need and get to the root of disease patterns.

Table 9.5 Poor memory

Efficacy of diamond	Diamonds support a coherent memory; they aid in reconstructing incidents and in retrieving information that you feel you know, but cannot recall.
Dosage	2–4 drops of the gem elixir, two times a day, or work out the daily dosage and add that to water, and sip the liquid all day long. Place a diamond on Yintang, the third eye. Note: Diamond strengthens the brain and also balances the corpus callosum, integrating the two hemispheres and their respective functions; for example, it can help with dyslexia.

Table 9.6 Stroke

Stroke	Aneurysm or cerebral thrombosis, embolism, hemorrhage, or sudden malfunction of blood circulation in the brain.
Signs and symptoms	Unconsciousness, paralysis, visual disturbances, loss of speech (aphasia), dizziness, severe headache, etc. If the attack is only a few minutes in duration, and the effects persist for only 24 hours, it is usually a transient ischemic attack (TIA), the origin of which may be arteriosclerosis, associated with high blood pressure, diabetes, etc.
Recommendations	Weight loss, physical exercise, no smoking or alcohol consumption, reduction of emotional stress, or a detoxification diet with appropriate nutrition—organic food, low amounts of animal protein, etc.
Efficacy of diamond	Works well after the stroke; integrate the diamond gem elixir with stroke treatments using needling and/or tuning forks. The acu-sound treatment is powerful and can help to ameliorate the deleterious effects immediately after an attack.
	Please note: if you feel that you have had a stroke, call an ambulance or emergency services immediately. Later you can incorporate the diamond gem elixir into your healing regimen.
	Note: Diamond gem elixir enhances the breakdown of blood clots and assists with the reorganization of the brain.
Dosage	3–7 drops of the gem elixir, three times a day; wait two weeks after the stroke.
Hildegard's gem therapy	More than 920 years ago, Hildegard was already aware of the connection between toxins and the waste products of human metabolism as they contributed to such conditions as gout and stroke, and she recommended her diamond white wine recipe (see Table 9.4). This gem water is not recommended until two weeks after a stroke.

Mars: Fire Element; Ruby

■ Mineral: Corundum; contains chromium

■ Planet: Mars; courageous, passionate, dynamic, decisive vs. aggressive, arrogant, cruel, impatient

GEM: RUBY

⬧ Spirit: Passion, confidence, hope, virtue

⬧ Mind: Dispels hopelessness (despair), depression, heartache

⬧ Body: Stimulates circulation, increases fever, raises blood pressure, treats adrenals, sexual organs, and back pain; natural painkiller

Syndromes: Specific Recommended Treatments

Table 9.7 Blood circulation

Efficacy of ruby	Helps with mild hypertension when used homeopathically. Being a powerful and robust crystal, it gives one courage and confidence in the face of any obstacle.
Dosage	5–7 drops of the ruby gem elixir, three times a day, or work out the daily dosage and add that to water, and sip the liquid all day long. Note: Ruby acts as a natural painkiller when placed on the site of pain, for example, the lower back, etc.

Table 9.8 Fever stimulant (febrifacient)

Efficacy of ruby	Ruby is a strong fever stimulant and can be applied or taken internally whenever fever is vital to the healing process. It supports the immune system and cleanses toxic waste substances from the body. The patient needs to rest, and drink water and herbal teas to offset the fluid loss due to perspiration.
Dosage	5–10 drops of the ruby gem elixir, three times a day, or work out the daily dosage and add that to water, and sip the liquid all day long. Place a ruby on the thymus gland, between the heart and the throat. If the fever rises too high, use cold compresses to reduce it, and do not continue with the Mars gem elixir; use the Saturn, which is cooling!

Table 9.9 Impotence

Impotence	Due to damage to the sexual organs, arterial blockage, diabetes mellitus, nerve damage to the spinal column, hormonal imbalance, heavy metal poisoning, medications, drugs, alcohol, and emotional imbalances
Efficacy of ruby	Treats impotence from emotional causes and general feeling of weakness. It encourages renewed passion and releases the fear of competition, failure, etc.
Dosage	3–7 drops of the ruby gem elixir, three times a day, or work out the daily dosage and add that to water, and sip the liquid all day long.

Mercury: Water Element; Lapis Lazuli

■ Mineral: Lazurite rock

■ Planet: Mercury; communication, creative intelligence, versatile vs. indecisive, opportunistic, restless, dishonest

Gem: Lapis Lazuli

◈ Spirit: Self-awareness, inner truth, wisdom, honesty; communicates freely

◈ Mind: Swallows anger and resentment, inability to express one's opinions

◈ Body: Throat, larynx/vocal cords, nerves, brain, thyroid

Syndromes: Specific Recommended Treatments

Table 9.10 Herpes

Herpes	Herpes is a virus that can lead to shingles, conjunctivitis, and infections in the genitals, etc. This treatment is only for herpes simplex virus 1: lip blisters.
Efficacy of lapis lazuli	Lapis lazuli gem elixir can be applied to the affected area to alleviate the burning sensation of herpes. Lemon balm (Melissa officialis essential oil) can be applied to the lip when there is a feeling of tightness or soreness; you can also use myrrh or tea tree essential oils.
Dosage	2–3 drops of the gem elixir per hour, or work out the daily dosage and add that to water, and sip the liquid all day long.

Table 9.11 Hoarseness

Hoarseness	Caused by an infection of the upper respiratory tract, colds, overuse of the voice, emotional issues, stage fright, nerves, overexcitement, suppressed anger, etc.
Efficacy of lapis lazuli	Lapis lazuli is used when anger is suppressed and there is difficulty verbalizing displeasure. It also treats strained, hoarse voices.
Dosage	3–7 drops of the gem elixir, three times per day, or work out the daily dosage and add that to water, and sip the liquid all day long. Wear as a pendant with the stone dangling near the Ren-22 Tiantu, throat area.
	Note: Lapis also treats loss of voice from hoarseness due to strained vocal cords, inflammation of the larynx, nerve disturbances in the vocal cords, polyps, vocal nodes, or loss of voice due to trauma. It also restores the voice quickly and facilitates the ability to raise the voice to speak one's truth.

Table 9.12 Hyper- and hypothyroidism

Efficacy of lapis lazuli	Lapis lazuli harmonizes both underactive and overactive thyroid glands.
Dosage	3–7 drops of the gem elixir, three times a day, or work out the daily dosage and add that to water, and sip the liquid all day long. Wear lapis as a necklace over Ren-22 Tiantu, the throat area.

Jupiter: Wood Element; Green Tourmaline

- ■ Mineral: Verdelite, boron, ring silicate

- ■ Planet: Jupiter; expansive, open, abundant, optimistic, tolerant, fortunate vs. indulgent, excessive, complacent

GEM: GREEN TOURMALINE

- ✦ Spirit: Grateful, open, understanding; embraces life

- ✦ Mind: Alleviates stress, anxiety, sorrow, frustration, bitterness

- ✦ Body: Effective for joint and nerve pain (analgesic), growth problems, scar therapy, impaired vision

SYNDROMES: SPECIFIC RECOMMENDED TREATMENTS

Table 9.13 Any degenerative diseases

Any degenerative diseases	These diseases manifest in the tissues, nerves, or joints, and are caused by deposits of waste products.
Efficacy of green tourmaline	Green tourmaline encourages purification and excretion of these substances. It also supports patience, the maintenance of an open mind, honesty, and sincerity.
Dosage	3–7 drops of the gem elixir, three times a day, or work out the daily dosage and add that to water, and sip the liquid all day long.

Table 9.14 Growth problems

Growth problems	The disruption of natural growth in children, which may be physiological, emotional, or congenital, or due to poor nutrition, illness, etc.
Efficacy of green tourmaline	Green tourmaline fosters the natural growth processes and overall development. TCM acknowledges that metabolic disturbances or malfunctions, and the associated loss of Qi, weaken the Wood element, which promotes normal growth and development.
Dosage	3–5 drops of the gem elixir, three times a day, or work out the daily dosage and add that to water, and sip the liquid all day long. Use the Eight Extraordinary meridian Du Mai as a treatment for stunted growth.

Table 9.15 Joint pains and problems

Joint pains and problems	Two factors need to be taken into consideration in the healing of joint pain and physical immobility—detoxification of the body and unrestricted circulation and blood flow to the extremities.
Efficacy of green tourmaline: Osteoarthritis	Green tourmaline is the most effective gem elixir for osteoarthritis, because it stimulates blood flow to the joints, reduces inflammation, and prevents the formation of degenerative damage. It also works psycho-emotionally, supports open-mindedness and flexible thinking, and lifts the spirits.
Dosage	5–7 drops of the gem elixir, three to five times a day, or work out the daily dosage and add that to water, and sip the liquid all day long.
Efficacy of green tourmaline. Rheumatoid arthritis	Green tourmaline is helpful in the early and progressive stages of rheumatism. It has several actions: • detoxifies, de-acidifies, and adjusts metabolism • reduces inflammation and pain • regenerates joints, muscles, and organs • emotionally addresses sadness and frustration, bitterness, and impatience • relieves pain.
Dosage	5–7 drops of the gem elixir, three to five times a day, or add the dosage to water, and sip the liquid all day long. For extreme pain, place a green tourmaline gem in front of a flashlight and use it as a gem "lens." Direct the refocused light at the affected area, three to seven times a day for 5–15 minutes.

Table 9.16 Scar therapy

Efficacy of green tourmaline	Green tourmaline stimulates Qi flow and alleviates the numbness associated with scars. It also heals severed nerves and improves the formation of nerves in the tissues.
Dosage	3–5 drops of the gem elixir, three times a day, or work out the daily dosage and add that to water, and sip the liquid all day long. For numbness: Place tourmaline rods on or near the affected area and point them away from the head, toward the hands and feet. For blocked Qi: Due to scar adhesions, for example, in a hysterectomy scar, point the gems upward on the front of the body, or downward on the back if the scar is located there. Note: Green tourmaline is a piezoelectric, dynamic, vibrant gem that can regenerate nerves and restore healthy functioning. Place gem rods on either side of the numb scar area during a treatment session.

Table 9.17 Vision problems

Efficacy of green tourmaline	Green tourmaline is used when vision is impaired by nerve damage; it also helps with squinting caused by nerve disturbances or injuries.
Dosage	5–9 drops of the gem elixir, three to five times a day, or work out the daily dosage and add that to water, and sip the liquid all day long.

Table 9.18 Synovitis

Synovitis	This occurs within the membranes surrounding the joint sinews and is an inflammatory, painful syndrome.
Efficacy of green tourmaline	Green tourmaline helps with both acute and chronic synovitis, no matter what the cause. It has a rapid analgesic effect on the tissue. It also regenerates tissue. Emotionally, it helps patients who need to control everything and believe that life is a constant struggle. The gem allows them to more easily accomplish their tasks and let things simply happen without effort.
Dosage	3–9 drops every hour for inflammation and pain, or work out the daily dosage and add that to water, and sip the liquid all day long.

Saturn: Earth Element; Blue Sapphire

■ Mineral: Corundum; aluminium oxide

■ Planet: Saturn; manifestation, patience, stability, perseverance, achievement, wisdom, self-discipline vs. rigidity, sorrow, delay, avarice, disappointment

GEM: BLUE SAPPHIRE

⬧ Spirit: Wisdom, inner calm, devotion, trust, goodwill, faith, ability to surrender, knowledge, concentration

⬧ Mind: Depression, stress, doubt, anger, impatience; natural antidepressant

⬧ Body: Relieves pain (analgesic), strengthens nerves, reduces fever and blood pressure

SYNDROMES: SPECIFIC RECOMMENDED TREATMENTS

Table 9.19 Stress, nerves, sexual harassment and abuse issues

Efficacy of blue sapphire	Blue sapphire tranquilizes the nerves, calms body/mind/spirit, and consequently treats immune deficiency caused by stress and abuse.
Dosage	3–5 drops of the gem elixir, three times a day, or work out the daily dosage and add that to water, and sip the liquid all day long.
Hildegard's gem therapy	Pour white wine over sapphires in a pitcher of water and sip all day long.

Table 9.20 Depression, insomnia

Efficacy of blue sapphire	According to Hildegard, blue sapphire is a natural antidepressant, is cooling and calming, and addresses issues of distrust and lack of faith in the self and the Divine. Patients who distrust life and have a dismal outlook about the future also may have insomnia.
Dosage	3–5 drops of the gem elixir, three times a day, and 3 drops at bedtime.
Hildegard's gem therapy	Place a blue sapphire over Yintang before retiring; this can also be taped in place overnight.

Table 9.21 Heartburn, gastritis, and digestion

Efficacy of blue sapphire	Blue sapphire addresses bitterness, sarcasm, anxiety, aggressiveness, impatience, and sudden anger, which can cause hyperacidity in the body and imbalances in the digestive system. It promotes kindness, goodwill, tolerance, open-mindedness, patience, and generosity with self and others.
Dosage	3–5 drops of the gem elixir, three times a day, or work out the daily dosage and add that to water, and sip the liquid all day long.
Hildegard's gem therapy	To confront sudden anger, stress, or impatience, place a tumbled larger sapphire in the mouth and hold it in place for five minutes.

Table 9.22 Lowers fever (febrifuge) and blood pressure

Efficacy of blue sapphire	The blue color of sapphire is cooling and the gem instills inner calm, quieting the body/mind/spirit, as well as lowering blood pressure and fever.
Dosage	3–7 drops of the gem elixir, three times a day, or work out the daily dosage and add that to water, and sip the liquid all day long. Also place cold compresses of this gem elixir under the calves and on the forehead and neck to reduce fever.

Table 9.23 As a general analgesic

Efficacy of blue sapphire	Blue sapphire can reduce inflammation and pain due to its quieting, cooling, calming, and grounding energy (qualities associated with Saturn).
Dosage	3–7 drops of the gem elixir, three to four times a day, or work out the daily dosage and add that to water, and sip the liquid all day long. Make a compress of the gem elixir and place on the pain. Place a section or slice of the stone over the painful area and shine a flashlight through the gem lens.

VibRadiance™ 5 Element Planetary Essential Oils ————

These organic and wildcrafted essential oil blends are also infused with gems. However, unlike the gem elixirs, the gemstones themselves have been introduced into, and remain in, the bottles to support the specific Five Element planetary profile on an archetypal and energetic level.

An innovative synergy of Chinese medicine principles, Five Element philosophy, Western astrological planetary archetypes, and gem and essential oil theory and lore has been utilized to produce these unique essential oil formulations. If you wish to have more details about each oil, i.e., the specific meridian involvement, contraindications, dermatological applications, associated constitutional imbalances, and psychological indications, please consult Mary Elizabeth's book *Constitutional Facial Acupuncture.*[8]

Please note that all the oils are blended in organic grapeseed and apricot seed carrier oils, plus vitamin E to ensure a longer shelf life and thereby prevent them from going rancid.

Each essential oil blend is categorized by the element, planetary personality, skin type, the infused gem and its qualities, and, of course, the various blended essential oils themselves.

Metal Element: Venus

This luscious essential oil blend represents love and beauty, the feminine principle, and embodiment of Aphrodite and Kuan Yin. It nourishes and enlivens the complexion, balances hormones and supports the Yin, calms the Shen mind, and promotes mindfulness.

- Planet: Venus appears in the heavens as a coruscating diamond, brilliant and welcoming, particularly in her light aspect as the Morning Star. Venus has a special relationship with Earth, in that they are virtually twin planets in their dimensions, and their orbital cycles involve them in a wonderfully graceful choreography that is beauty and elegance personified.

- Usage: This oil is beneficial for dry and mature skin, because the component oils contain phytoestrogens.

- Gem: The gem infused in this oil blend is white quartz, which reflects the color of the Metal element, and the harmonizing and relational aspects of these goddesses.

- Oils: Rose otto, geranium, ylang-ylang, yarrow, thyme, lemongrass, etc.

Fire Element: Mars

This spicy blend represents the masculine principle, courage, the ability to be dynamic, and the explosive energy of the zodiacal sign Aries. It supports the adrenals, unblocks sinus congestion, stimulates digestion, lessens anxiety, and preserves the beauty and integrity of the skin.

- Planet: Since time immemorial, Mars has cast its baleful red glare upon Earth, reminding us of the very worst of our human nature, our capacity for violence and self-destruction. Properly the domicile of various bellicose, warlike gods, its scarlet tinge is echoed in the blood that is shed in time of war, yet it also represents the capacity for us to channel our passion in acts of beneficent creation, and assert ourselves in a life-affirming way without aggression or malice.

- Usage: This blend enlivens dull, lifeless skin, addresses bruises, acne, and dermatitis, and can decrease inflammation. Be careful not to apply it to sensitive, dry skin!

- Gem: Red garnet promotes courage, passion, and action; its red hue represents blood, the warrior, and the Fire element.

- Oils: Ginger, myrrh, basil, black pepper, helichrysum, cumin, pine, etc.

Water Element: Mercury

This multifaceted blend represents creativity and communication, Mercury, the Quicksilver Messenger, and the adaptable energy of Hermes. It lessens age spots and scars, softens wrinkles, promotes longevity, quiets the nerves, and eases the heart.

- Planet: Mercury/Hermes, the Trickster, is of that special class of deities whose attentions may or may not be welcome. The avatars of this archetype may not always be the most scrupulous of individuals, but they also possess the capacity to alter the nature of reality through their creative engagement with the truth,[9] and they facilitate communication between different realms of experience, in the same manner as the Quicksilver Messenger, who traveled from Olympus to Hades at the behest of Zeus.

◈ Usage: This essential oil formulation treats oily, dry, and mature skin; as a cellular regenerator, it is especially recommended for sagging skin, wrinkles, hyperpigmentation, and scars.

◈ Gem: Blue lapis lazuli represents the Water Element; this stone facilitates communication of all kinds, heightens awareness, and reflects the creativity and vibrancy of the psychopomp Mercury.

◈ Oils: Clary sage, lavender, carrot seed, rosemary verbonne, fennel, bergamot, etc.

Wood Element: Jupiter

This expansive blend represents joy and abundance, the optimistic deity Jupiter, and the powerful energy of Zeus, the King of the Olympian gods! It promotes sensuality, eases childbirth, aids in weight loss, and treats burns and likewise Kidney and respiratory imbalances.

◈ Planet: The largest of all the planets, and according to astronomers, a failed sun, archetypal Jupiter permits us to engage with the world with optimism and insight. Its avuncular bonhomie and goodwill facilitate our enjoyment of the manifold blessings in life, lending a singular spirit to our everyday endeavors.

◈ Usage: When using this blend, hormones are balanced, optimism reigns, and depression is banished. Skin issues like broken capillaries and acne are ameliorated; it also helps with labor pains and weight loss.

◈ Gem: Green aventurine relates to the Gall Bladder and Liver; it allows the patient to cultivate an easygoing, loving nature, qualities that are associated with Jupiter.

◈ Oils: Jasmine, sage, grapefruit, clove, Roman chamomile, balsam fir, etc.

Earth Element: Saturn

This cooling, astringent essential oil blend represents the qualities patience and perseverance, the capacity to manifest, and the sage Saturn/ Chronos, the Time-Keeper. It addresses edema, cools heat, increases the libido, encourages the memory, and supports the process of grieving. Saturn, like Mercury, possesses properties of cellular regeneration.

- Planet: The coldest and darkest of the traditional planets, Saturn is traditionally associated with death, and it is particularly appropriate for the treatment of grief associated with loss. Saturn is the Taskmaster, who imposes its strictures upon the material world, engendering obstacles that may temporarily hinder us in our forward progress, but which ultimately are to our benefit.

- Usage: The Saturn blend is excellent for mature skin, and the treatment of hot flashes and red face due to menopause or hypertension. It regenerates the skin, promotes both masculine and feminine libido, calms nervous tension, and, consistent with its Earth element associations, promotes grounding.

- Gem: Yellow citrine fosters abundance, aids digestion, treats birth trauma, and facilitates the manifestation of one's dreams in the world.

- Oils: Cypress, cumin, Atlas cedar, frankincense, galbanum, bergamot, etc.

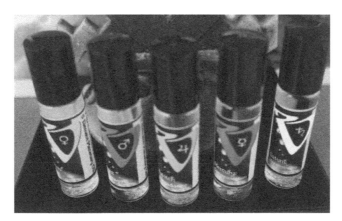

Figure 9.3 *VibRadiance™ 5 Element Planetary Essential Oils*

Treatment Recommendations

The VibRadiance™ 5 Element Planetary Essential Oils come in a large 2 oz size and smaller ⅓ oz roller bottles that can conveniently be rolled upon acupuncture and/or acu-sound points. This is a highly effective way to address Five Element planetary disharmonies even without stimulating the points in question with needles or tuning forks. For example, you can apply the 5 Element Planetary Essential Oil appropriate to a given point using the roller bottles to enhance the results of the treatments; this is particularly useful when treating the Eight Extraordinary meridians (see Chapter 3), as suggested here:

- Chong Mai, Earth: Sp-4 Gongsun, Grandfather/Grandson (Saturn)

- Yin Wei Mai, Fire: PC-6 Neiguan, Inner Pass (Mars)

- Ren Mai, Metal: Lu-7 Lieque, Broken Sequence (Venus)

- Yin Qiao Mai, Water: Kid-6 Zhaohai, Shining Sea (Mercury)

- Du Mai, Fire: SI-3 Houxi, Back Stream (Mars)

- Yang Qiao Mai, Water: Bl-62 Shenmai, Extending Vessel (Mercury)

- Dai Mai, Wood: GB-41 Zulinqi, Foot Governor of Tears (Jupiter)

- Yang Wei Mai, Fire: TH-5 Waiguan, Outer Pass (Mars).

These roller bottles may be used on other acupuncture points and acu-sound points anywhere else on the body, for example:

- the Source Luo points (see Chapter 4)

- the Five Element vibrational hara points (see Chapter 7)

- solo sound therapy (see Chapter 8): the Sacred Mudra Ritual

- the Grounding Protocol points (see Chapter 8).

Usage of the VibRadiance™ 5 Element Planetary Essential Oils enhances the Qi and adds a new dimension to your vibrational treatments.

Please note: Make sure that your patient is not allergic to essential oils in general, or to any individual oil found in the planetary blends you are considering using. Do test them for sensitivity prior to treatment. Some people are allergic to the scent of these oils when diffused in the air. Smell is the most ancient sensory faculty we possess, and it acts upon the limbic, reptilian brain. Even if an individual patient isn't allergic, there may yet be unpleasant memories associated with certain scents. For example, you might have had a British grandmother who, without your consent, placed sprigs of fresh lavender in your underwear drawer to keep your "knickers" fresh. You don't particularly cherish your grandmother, and thus the smell of lavender essential oil conjures up these unpleasant recollections.

In order to test for sensitivity, apply the oil or blend to the inside of the person's forearm a minimum of 12 hours before using it elsewhere on the body. You should also ensure that they will not react to any oils diffused in the air.

Crème Vitale ESP Rose: An Organic Moisturizing Cream with Bulgarian Rose Essential Oil

This lush, non-greasy cream contains the hydrating, phytoestrogenic qualities of the precious essential oil Bulgarian rose, coupled with the Shen-balancing antioxidant action of pearl powder. Psychospiritually, Bulgarian rose promotes well-being and self-acceptance, and opens the Heart.

Ingredients
Bulgarian Rose, *Rosa Damascena*, Mi Gui Hua
Rose otto essential oil is an antidepressant, a nervine, a stimulant, a hormone balancer, an aphrodisiac, and an emmenagogue, which can initiate menstruation, therefore it is contraindicated during pregnancy. It regenerates mature, dry skin, treats sensitive skin, and is effective in alleviating symptoms of eczema and broken capillaries.

As it possesses phytoestrogenic attributes, constitutionally, it can ease the discomfort of menopause and PMS. On a psychospiritual level, it uplifts emotions, and treats depression, exhaustion, stress, and shock by supporting the Yin.

Pearl Powder, *Margarita*, Zhen Zhu

Pearl powder has been used in China for centuries to brighten the complexion, sharpen vision, reduce redness, even out blotchy or discolored skin (hyperpigmentation), and encourage the healing of burns, wounds, and mouth ulcers. It contains a high amount of calcium, which accelerates the healing process.

Internally, it can be ingested to address syndromes like insomnia, palpitations, and irritability. Externally, due to the presence of silica, pearl powder can prevent skin aging, and it is beneficial for the maintenance of healthy hair, nails, and teeth.

Organic sunflower seed (*Helianthus annuus*) oil

Organic sunflower seed oil is a natural emollient, which contains:

- 82 percent oleic acid, which mirrors the sebum (natural oils) of the skin

- antioxidant omega-6 (linoleic acid)

- a high vitamin E and squalene content.

Organic white willow bark (*Salix alba*)

Organic white willow bark contains salicylic acid, which is the natural, original herbal source for this active ingredient of the drug aspirin. Willow bark gently exfoliates the skin, closes the pores, and lessens the appearance of fine lines and wrinkles, protecting the skin from environmental pollutants.

It contains:

- flavonoids

- tannins

- powerful antioxidants.

Organic neem seed oil (*Azadirachta indica*)

Organic neem seed oil has:

- antiseptic properties

- linoleic and oleic acids.

It is used for skin disorders in traditional Ayurvedic medicine, and treats acne, eczema, and inflammation.

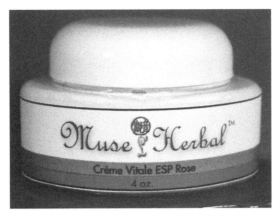

Figure 9.4 *Crème Vitale ESP Rose*

Three Essential Oil Hydrosols

A hydrosol is the aromatic water that remains after the distillation of an essential oil, either by steam or water. We refer to them by a variety of names—hydrosols, hydrolates, or distillates. Floral waters usually are not a product of a distillation process; rather, the essential oils contained in them have simply been added to water. Consequently, these floral waters possess neither the therapeutic properties of the plant, nor the exquisite aroma.[10]

Lavender Hydrosol (Lavandula Angustifolia)

The organic lavender hydrosol is cooling and clears heat from the head, reduces facial redness, treats blocked sinuses caused by Liver Qi stagnation and treats sun-damaged skin, burns, scarring, and Shen disturbances.

Bulgarian Rose Hydrosol (Rosa Damascena)

Bulgarian rose is phytoestrogenic, hence it nourishes the Yin, moisturizes dry skin, balances hormones, and lessens hot flashes, irritability, and depression, calms the Shen, and communicates with the Heart, both physically and emotionally.

Neroli Hydrosol (Citrus Aurantium)

Neroli has euphoric qualities, clears Heart fire, relieves stress, depression, insomnia, and palpitations, and treats all skin conditions.

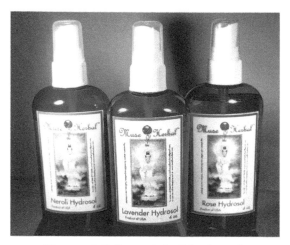

Figure 9.5 *Essential oil hydrosols*

A Recommended Treatment Protocol

At this juncture, you, the practitioner, have been introduced to a great deal of information concerning treatment protocols and vibrational remedies. We have additionally made suggestions as to the best way to integrate the two modalities, acupuncture needling and tuning forks, into your Vibrational Acupuncture™ treatments for patients, or as a self-treatment regimen.

Here is a suggested course of treatment that we feel would be most effective for you to implement in your practice; we have also pointed out optional protocols that you may wish to integrate later into your treatment sessions.

1. Always begin with the Grounding Protocol and the Corpus Callosum Balancing treatment (see Chapter 8). Optional: The Sacred Mudra Ritual (see Chapter 8). Remember to use only tuning forks in these treatments.

2. Use master/couple points for the Eight Extraordinary meridians with Fascia Talk. Optional: The Earth glyph and Sound Tube treatments (see Chapter 3).

3. Treat Source Luo constitutional points for emotional imbalances and/or physical exhaustion. Optional: The Twister, "V" Vortex, and Three Treasures treatments (see Chapter 4).

4. Integrate motor/trigger points into an effective temporomandibular joint dysfunction (TMJ) treatment. Optional: Muscle release points for the neck and shoulders. Both tuning forks and/or acupuncture points can be utilized (see Chapter 5).

5. Perform the Vibrational Balancing Facial Protocol with only tuning forks (see Chapter 6). Optional: Address a sagging neck with the motor points for the platysma muscle, using tuning forks and/or needles (see Chapter 6).

6. Practice palpating the hara, and then choose one relevant Five Element treatment per patient (see Chapter 7); tuning forks are suggested. Optional: Needles.

Other Considerations

The chakra-balancing treatments in this chapter, particularly those with the donut gems and the related acupuncture points, will be very useful for you. You can combine them with the Grounding Protocol, resonating the Acutonics Ohm® Unison combination through the hole in the center of the appropriate donut gem; if you're unsure as to how to accomplish this, do examine the treatment photos in this chapter.

Do make use of the 5 Element Planetary Gem Elixirs, both topically and internally; you can drop them on acu-sound treatment points. The 5 Element Planetary Essential Oil roller bottles (⅓ oz) are very effective on the master/couple points of the Eight Extraordinary meridians, the Source Luo emotional points, and the chakra points. Use your imagination and be creative.

As we have noted, the gem elixirs are powerfully effective when ingested to address Five Element planetary disharmonies; please note the disclaimer and adhere to the indicated dosages.

When you're working on the face, we recommend that you massage in our *Crème Vitale ESP Rose* moisturizing cream, and conclude your treatment with one of the three essential oil hydrosols, depending upon the needs of your patient.

Reminder: Always thoroughly ground yourself prior to the beginning of each treatment; this will help you stay focused and clear, and facilitate greater ease in making an appropriate decision about which treatments to feature in a given session. Sometimes, just listening to the Ohm tone will engender deeper, more grounded breathing and reconnect you to the Source. You can also treat the master/couple points of the Dai Mai, which will similarly provide greater clarity.

The information and treatment protocols in this book are the product of many years of teaching and experimenting with a wide range of approaches; we want to encourage you in your exploration of this exciting new aspect of your practice, Vibrational Acupuncture™!

Chapter 10

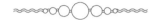

A Personal Note from
the Authors

*To accomplish great things, we must not only act, but also dream;
not only plan, but also believe.*

Anatole France

As you have undoubtedly surmised, there is nothing comparable to this book, *Vibrational Acupuncture: Integrating Tuning Forks with Needles*. There are books that instruct the reader in the use of various types of tuning forks, and other books which provide instruction in the proper employment of acupuncture needles, but no one textbook has offered strategies for the integration of the two, a marriage of Venus and Mars.

In the previous nine chapters, we have progressively outlined our philosophy and provided you with original treatment protocols to facilitate your implementation of both modalities. We have included helpful diagrams, tables of useful information, and high-quality treatment photographs, so as to render the details of the various treatments sufficiently clear that you may successfully integrate them within your established practice or apply them in self-treatment.

Please note that all of these protocols have been tested by us throughout our years of teaching, as well as in private practice. This unique synergy of tuning forks with acupuncture needling initiates a powerful transformational process of healing.

Some Caveats and Cautions

- If you are not a licensed or registered (or otherwise qualified) acupuncturist, do not attempt to treat anyone, including yourself, with acupuncture needles. Your lack of understanding of the modality could cause harm to yourself or others.

- If a therapist has not been trained in acupuncture and Chinese medicine, do not book an appointment with them. Invest time in seeking out a licensed/registered, etc., practitioner who has completed three-plus years of training in an accredited acupuncture school. Avoid booking an appointment with a practitioner who is not a qualified acupuncturist. If you're not sure as to a given practitioner's level of expertise, do not hesitate to make inquiries about their credentials—how long they studied and what degree they received. Documents attesting to this should be readily displayed in their offices.

- Do not mistake "dry needling" for acupuncture; there is no such comparison to be made. A needle is either a hypodermic needle that is used to inject medication or it is an acupuncture needle, a filiform, thread-like needle. "Dry" needles are simply acupuncture needles.

Some Recommendations

- Whether you are an acupuncturist, sound healer, or other professional—or a layperson—do feel free to use the Acutonics Ohm® Unison tuning forks for any and all of the recommended sound healing protocols in this book. If you are interested in purchasing these forks for your practice, you may contact us at *Chi-Akra Center for Ageless Aging* for details or order them directly from the Acutonics® website: www.acutonics.com.

- To date, there are no regulatory bodies for sound healing in the US (and, to the best of our knowledge, internationally, as well), so you may feel free to explore this exciting modality without fear of reprisal, oversight, or censure.

◈ Just as a reminder, this book contains a range of protocols that do not require acupuncture needles.

◈ If you wish to learn more from us about sound healing, we would welcome your participation in future seminars in *Facial Soundscapes*™. We do offer a certification to those practitioners who complete all five modules of training.

◈ The tuning fork protocols presented in Chapter 8 are especially wonderful for super-sensitive patients and will be equally effective as part of a self-healing regimen.

- The Grounding Protocol: very few people in our culture are sufficiently grounded or have healing contact with nature.

- The Sacred Mudra Ritual: Lacing the Three Jiaos

  – The Pyramid Position

  – The Prayer Position

  – The Inner Child Position.

- The Corpus Callosum Balancing treatment: to harmonize the twin hemispheres of the brain. These days, as we have extensively documented elsewhere in the book, everyone's linear left brain is overtaxed by their constant interface with electronic devices.

◈ Do review the contents of Chapter 2, relating to practical discernment, i.e., whether to use tuning forks or needles.

- Make a note of the benefits and contraindications for both modalities.

- Review the contraindicated points for pregnancy which apply to each modality; these points induce the onset of labor.

Some Things to Remember

◈ The vibrational Qi of tuning forks is an adaptogen; when your patient has absorbed sufficient resonance, you will note that the sound is no longer traveling into their body, and you will feel it in your wrists or arms. This feedback is something that is not afforded by other modalities, i.e., microcurrent, laser, etc., and provides you with greater insight into the patient's state during the treatment. When you discern that no further sound is being transmitted, your patient is "cooked," and the vibrations are, instead, being taken in by you. At this point, you can move on to the next set of points, etc., or stop the treatment.

◦ We encourage you to set aside time to read this book at a leisurely pace so that you may absorb the information gradually; however, do focus on what is important for you at the moment.

Just as a reminder, here is a brief recap of each chapter and its content.

Introduction: This chapter contains a great deal of important information about Chinese medicine, how the ancient Chinese (and others) perceived sound, and how the influence of music that was less than "upright" contributed to the ultimate demise of the Chinese Empire in 1912.

Chapter 1: This chapter presents some rudimentary concepts of music theory, and an atomic paradigm of sound vibration, which may be easier to understand. It is an attempt to provide you with a basic understanding of the nature of sound vibrations as they are employed in the various tuning fork protocols. Even if you don't understand it, read it in its entirety; you will learn important information about the nature and use of musical intervals, particularly the unison and the octave, ideas of consonance vs. dissonance, etc.

Chapter 3: This chapter addresses the Eight Extraordinary meridians, our pre-natal Qi and genetic blueprint.

◦ It introduces the concept and practice of "Fascia Talk," providing you with a means to discern the master point of these channels by palpation, which is an excellent tool for non-acupuncturists.

◦ The material presented on psychospiritual aspects of the Eight Extraordinary vessels is unique, offering perspectives beyond those traditionally associated with these all-important channels.

◦ Do incorporate the treatments based on sacred geometry:

• Earth Glyph

- The Figure 8/Infinity Symbol

- The Sound Tube.

Chapter 4: This chapter on anti-exhaustion treatments addresses postnatal Qi and lifestyle choices.

- Source/Luo treatments for emotional issues

- Sacred geometry treatments:

  - The Twister

  - The "V" Vortex

  - The Three Treasures.

- We conclude with a consideration of the worldwide phenomenon of the "hypertrophy" of the eye. As sound healing practitioners, it is crucial for you to understand the difference between the two ways of perceiving reality and how the dominance of the eye over the ear is refashioning our culture in ways that are detrimental to our well-being. "The eye judges, and is aggressive; the ear compares and is receptive."[1]

Chapters 5 and 6: Both chapters introduce the use of motor points for various purposes:

- temporomandibular joint dysfunction (TMJ)

- palpation techniques

- a facial balancing treatment (tuning forks only)

- a motor point treatment for sagging neck (platysma muscle).

Chapter 7: This chapter provides a comprehensive overview of Japanese hara diagnosis, featuring the Five Elements, techniques of abdominal palpation, and treatments using both modalities.

Chapter 9: The use of the vibrational and topical treatments in this chapter will enhance the results of other protocols.

- Comprehensive information has been provided regarding the use of gem elixirs, and a *materia medica* presenting remedies drawn from the medical writings of 12th century abbess, Hildegard of

Bingen is included; we have similarly catalogued information concerning our own QuintEssentials™ line of 5 Element Planetary Gem Elixirs, which have produced remarkable results in treatments in our seminars and private practice. Do read the various illustrative anecdotes.

⊕ Our VibRadiance™ 5 Element Planetary Essential Oils can be used effectively in treatments for both face and body; these potent essential oil blends can be applied directly to Five Element acupuncture points in lieu of needling or be used as an adjunct for needle insertions (around the point) or directly on the point (tuning forks).

⊕ Our luscious *Crème Vitale ESP Rose* moisturizing cream, infused with organic Bulgarian rose essential oil and pearl powder, will enhance the results of the facial treatments presented in Chapter 6.

⊕ Spritz organic essential oil hydrosols (Bulgarian rose, neroli, and lavender) can be used on the face at the conclusion of a treatment.

⊕ Donut gems can be laid upon the body over acupuncture points and chakra locations, and needled or forked through.

A Final Word

We hope that you will feel free to explore this new territory, this *terra incognita*, for yourself and your patients. There are always risks involved in striking forth in unprecedented directions, but we want to assure you that we are available at all times (unless we're teaching, traveling or sleeping, or perhaps writing another book!) to answer questions and provide recommendations for incorporating these transformative treatment protocols as part of your existing practice or to further your own journey of self-transformation.

Our separate life and career trajectories have led us, unswervingly, in the last 27 years to the pursuit of healing and mentorship through teaching. At heart, however, we remain singers and performers... This is an aspect of our joint biography which we cannot, and would not, forsake. A singer who strives for the highest level of artistic expression must become a listener *par excellence.*

Latterly, we have brought these refined listening skills to bear upon all aspects of our lives—our healing work, our teaching, our creative efforts, separate and collective, musical and otherwise, as well as our relationship. We hope that you, too, will learn to turn an attentive ear to the world around you, shutting out the manifold distractions of the restless eye, and find, in the stillness at the eye of the storm, the immortality that is present in every waking moment:

It is as though he listened
and such listening as his enfolds us in silence
in which at last we begin to hear
what we are meant to be.

Lao-Tzu

Mary Elizabeth Wakefield, L.Ac., M.S., M.M.
MichelAngelo, M.F.A., C.T.M.
Chi-Akra Center for Ageless Aging
New York, NY
www.facialacupuncture-wakefieldtechnique.com and chi.akra@gmail.com

Endnotes

Acknowledgements

1   Wakefield, Mary Elizabeth (2014) *Constitutional Facial Acupuncture*. London: Churchill Livingstone Elsevier.
2   Carey, Donna *et al.* (2010) *Acutonics from Galaxies to Cells: Planetary Science, Harmony and Medicine*. Llano, NM: Devachan Press.

Introduction

1   OUP (2013) *Oxford English Dictionary* (11th edition). Oxford: Oxford University Press.
2   A neuropeptide is a "vasopressin, and a nine-amino-acid peptide secreted by the nerve endings in the neural lobe of the pituitary... It secretes substance P, a major bioactive peptide in many neural pathways, including pain signaling." Mains, Richard and Eipper, Betty A. (1999) *The Neuropeptides*. Philadelphia, PA: Lippincott-Raven.
3   Gaynor, Mitchell L. (2002) *The Healing Power of Sound: Recovery from Life-Threatening Illness using Sound, Voice and Music*. Boston, MA: Shambhala Publications, p.33.
4   Jespersen, Otto (2016) *Language, Its Nature, Development and Origin*. Palala Press.
5   Mithen, Steven (2006) *The Singing Neanderthals: The Origins of Music, Language, Mind and Body*. Cambridge, MA: Harvard University Press, p.221.
6   Schneider, Achim (2014) "Ice-age musicians fashioned ivory flute." Accessed on April 24, 2019 at www.nature.com/news/2004/041213/full/041213-14.html.
7   Sigerson, John and Wolfe, Kathy (1992) *A Manual on the Rudiments of Tuning and Registration. Book 1: Introduction and Human Singing Voice*. Washington, DC: Schiller Institute (Kindle version).
8   This overt and uninhibited expression of intense emotion, similar to that invoked by a Greek chorus, gives the family and friends permission to vent their own emotions in the present moment, which facilitates the necessary process of detachment and healing.
9   Brindley, Erica Fox (2012) *Music, Cosmology and the Politics of Harmony in Early China*. Albany, NY: SUNY Press, pp.4–5.
10 *Ibid.*, p.134; from Yang, *Chunqiu Zuozhuan zhu*, 10.1.12, 1221–22.
11 Empedocles also proposed the existence of two great organizing principles within the universe, Love and Strife, which are analogous to the Chinese Yin and Yang.
12 Apel, Willi (1968) *Harvard Dictionary of Music*. Cambridge, MA: Harvard University Press, p.137.
13 Wu, Zhongxian and Wu, Karen (2014) *Heavenly Stems and Earthly Branches—TianGan DiZhi: The Heart of Chinese Wisdom Traditions*. London: Singing Dragon, p.40.
14 *Ibid.*, p.138; citing Xiong, Xunzi, *Winged Diversity*, p.415 (translated by Cook).
15 Apel, *op. cit.*, p.136.
16 Tame, David (1984) *The Secret Power of Music: The Transformation of Self and Society through Musical Energy*. Rochester, VT: Destiny Books, p.57.
17 *Ibid.*, p.51.

Chapter 1

1   Although, as was indicated in the Introduction, tuning forks produce very little in the way of overtones; this is perhaps advantageous in a therapeutic context, as the tones utilized by the practitioner who uses the Acutonics® tuning forks represent the purest distillation of the planetary essence.
2   In fact, there is a precise formula for determining the maximum number of electrons in a given shell, which is $2n^2$ (where n = the number of the energy shell); this gives us maximum numbers of

electrons for the first four shells of 2, 8, 18, and 32, respectively. Jefferson Lab (n.d.) "Questions and Answers." Accessed on April 25, 2019 at https://education.jlab.org/qa/electron_number.html.

3 Sigerson, John and Wolfe, Kathy (1992) *A Manual on the Rudiments of Tuning and Registration. Book 1: Introduction and Human Singing Voice.* Washington, DC: Schiller Institute (Kindle version).

4 Koestler, Arthur (2017) *The Sleepwalkers: A History of Man's Changing View of the Universe.* London: Penguin Arkana.

5 *Ibid.*

6 Hetherington, Norriss S. (Ed.) (2014) *Encyclopedia of Cosmology (Routledge Revivals): Historical, Philosophical, and Scientific Foundations of Modern Cosmology.* New York, NY: Routledge.

7 James, Jamie (1995) *The Music of the Spheres: Music, Science and the Natural Order of the Universe.* New York, NY: Copernicus Books, pp.30–31.

8 Rudhyar, Dane (1982) *The Magic of Tone and the Art of Music.* Boston, MA: Shambhala Books.

9 Taylor, T. (translator) (1818) *Iamblichus' Life of Pythagoras or Pythagoric Life.* London: J.M. Watkins, p.60.

10 See Guthrie, Kenneth Sylvan (translator and compiler) (1988) *The Pythagorean Sourcebook and Library.* Grand Rapids, MI: Phanes Press.

11 That is, the intervals of the unison, the perfect 5th and the perfect 4th.

12 Taylor, T. (translator) (1818) *Iamblichus' Life of Pythagoras or Pythagoric Life.* London: J.M. Watkins, p.62.

13 Ferguson, Kitty (2008) *The Music of Pythagoras: How an Ancient Brotherhood Cracked the Code of the Universe and Lit the Path from Antiquity to Outer Space.* New York, NY: Walker & Company, p.67.

14 Tame, David (1984) *The Secret Power of Music: The Transformation of Self and Society through Musical Energy.* Rochester, VT: Destiny Books, p.204.

15 Sigerson and Wolfe, *op. cit.* LaRouche's article, which originally appeared in *Executive Intelligence Review 18*, 1, 1991, is reprinted as the foreword to this book.

16 Voss, Angela (n.d.) *The Music of the Spheres: Ficino and Renaissance Harmonia.* Accessed on April 29, 2019 at http://gnosticacademy.com/voss-a-the-music-of-the-spheres-ficino-and-renaissance-harmonia/.

17 *Ibid.*

18 Tame, *op. cit.*, p.239.

19 Cousto, Hans (2000) *The Cosmic Octave: Origin of Harmony.* Mendocino, CA: Life Rhythm Publications, p.10.

20 Campbell, Joseph (1964) *The Masks of God: Occidental Mythology, Volume 3.* New York, NY: Viking Press, pp.21–22.

21 Kerenyi, Carl (1951) *The Gods of the Greeks.* London: Thames & Hudson, p.18.

22 Sjöö, Monica and Mor, Barbara (1991) *The Great Cosmic Mother: Rediscovering the Religion of the Earth.* San Francisco, CA: Harper San Francisco, p.63.

23 See, e.g., Gimbutaus, Marija (2001) *The Language of the Goddess.* London: Thames & Hudson and Walker, Barbara (1983) *The Woman's Encyclopedia of Myths and Secrets.* New York, NY: HarperCollins Publishers.

24 Jung, Carl (1962) *Memories, Dreams, Reflections.* New York, NY: Pantheon Books. An excerpt from his memoir, accessed on 28 May, 2019 at www.near-death.com/experiences/notable/carl-jung.html.

25 However, it can certainly be argued that the average musical listener of the early 21st century is comfortable with a much greater level of comparative dissonance than their medieval or Renaissance counterpart.

26 Meyer, Kathi (1952) "The Eight Gregorian Modes on the Cluny Capitals." *Art Bulletin 34*, 2, 75–94. Although the inscription is describing the eighth Gregorian church mode, it arguably applies also to the octave.

Chapter 2

1 Kaptchuk, Ted (1983) *The Web That Has No Weaver: Understanding Chinese Medicine.* Chicago, IL: Congdon and Weed, p.43.

2 McTaggart, Lynne (2007) *The Intention Experiment: The Transformation of Self and Society through Musical Energy.* Rochester, VT New York, NY: Free Press, p.xxv.

3 University of Washington (2001) "Brains of Deaf People Rewire to 'Hear' Music." *ScienceDaily.* Accessed on April 29, 2019 at www.sciencedaily.com/releases/2001/11/011128035455.htm.

4 Gray, John (1992) *Men Are from Mars, Women Are from Venus: The Classic Guide to Understanding the Opposite Sex.* New York, NY: HarperCollins Publishers.

Chapter 3

1 Wakefield, Mary Elizabeth (2014) *Constitutional Facial Acupuncture.* London: Churchill Livingstone Elsevier, p.30.

2 Keown, Daniel (2014) *The Spark in the Machine: How the Science of Acupuncture Explains the Mysteries of Western Medicine.* London: Singing Dragon, p.10.

3 *Ibid.*, p.11.

4 Wakefield, *op. cit.*, pp.27–28.

5   BEC Crew (2016) "Scientists just captured the flash of light that sparks when a sperm meets an egg." Accessed on April 31, 2019 at www.sciencealert.com/scientists-just-captured-the-actual-flash-of-light-that-sparks-when-sperm-meets-an-egg. It should be noted, however, that this phenomenon has only been observed under laboratory conditions, not *in vivo*.

6   Shlain, Leonard (2004) *Sex, Time and Power: How Women's Sexuality Shaped Human Evolution*. New York, NY: Penguin Books.

Chapter 4

1   Deadman, Peter, Al-Khafaji, Mazin, and Baker, Kevin (1998) *A Manual of Acupuncture*. London: Journal of Chinese Medicine Publications, p.39.

2   Wilde, Oscar, from his play *Lady Windermere's Fan*.

3   Berendt, Joachim-Ernst (1992) *The Third Ear: On Listening to the World*. New York, NY: Henry Holt and Co., p.27.

4   Berendt, Joachim-Ernst (1987) *Nada Brahma: The World Is Sound; Music and the Landscape of Consciousness*. New York, NY: Henry Holt and Co., p.6.

5   A good example of this is Gustav Klimt's famous 1907 painting of Adele Bloch-Bauer, recently celebrated in the movie *Woman in Gold*. This outstanding work of art, commissioned by Ms. Bauer and her husband from the artist, was stolen by the Nazis during World War II, and eventually was relocated by a descendant. The painting was later acquired by Ronald Lauder from the family for 135 million dollars!

6   Berendt (1992), *op. cit.*, p.53.

7   Voss, Angela (n.d.) *The Theurgic Symbol: Musico-Magic Therapeutics in the Sixteenth Century*, p.1. Accessed on April 30, 2019 at www.academia.edu/32728827/Music_and_Magic.

8   Berendt (1987) *op. cit.*, p.27.

9   *Ibid.*, p.5.

10   Fottrell, Quentin (2018) "People spend most of their waking hours staring at screens." Accessed on 21 August, 2019 at https://www.marketwatch.com/story/people-are-spending-most-of-their-waking-hours-staring-at-screens-2018-08-01.

11   Carr, Nicholas (2011) *The Shallows: What the Internet Is Doing to Our Brains*. New York, NY: W. W. Norton & Company.

12   *Ibid.* p.16 (Kindle version).

13   *Ibid.*

14   Alpha rhythms are a pattern of slow brain waves (alpha waves) in normal persons at rest with closed eyes, thought by some to be associated with an alert but daydreaming mind.

Chapter 5

1   Travell, Janet G. and Simons, David G. (1983) *Myofascial Pain and Dysfunction: The Trigger Point Manual, Volume 1*. Baltimore, MD: Williams & Wilkins, p.223.

Chapter 6

1   The first episode of season 3 of the British sci-fi series *Black Mirror*, entitled "Nosedive," extrapolated from this aspect of online existence to postulate a society where everyone was constantly being rated by others, using phones and *optical* implants. The accumulation of quasi-Facebook "likes" from this battery of strangers was essential to the maintenance of one's status in the culture at large.

2   Tsay, Chia-Jung (2013) "Sight over sound in the judgment of music performance." *Proceedings of the National Academy of Sciences 110*, 36, 14580–14585.

3   Another highly prescient sci-fi television series from the 1960s, Rod Serling's *Twilight Zone*, featured a memorable episode entitled "Number 12 Looks Just Like You." In a future utopia, at a certain age, each citizen, regardless of appearance, was presented with the societally sanctioned option of having their consciousness transplanted into a number of limited, but highly attractive, physical somatotypes. The heroine of the episode, an average-looking young girl, initially resisted the allure of such idealized perfection and the loss of her personal identity, but eventually submitted to the procedure.

Chapter 7

1   García, Héctor and Miralles, Francesc (2017) *Ikigai: The Japanese Secret to a Long and Happy Life* (translated by Cleary Heather). New York, NY: Penguin Books.

2   Matsumoto, Kiiko and Birch, Stephen (1988) *Hara Diagnosis: Reflections on the Sea*. Brookline, MA: Paradigm Publications.

3   Denmei, Shudo (2011) *Introduction to Meridian Therapy*. Seattle WA: Eastland Press, p.88.

4   Kiiko and Stephen, *op. cit.*, p24.

5   *Ibid.*, p.25.

6   *Ibid.*

7   *Ibid.*, p.275.

8   Kaptchuk, Ted (1983) *The Web That Has No Weaver: Understanding Chinese Medicine*. Chicago, IL: Congdon & Weed, p.343.

9   Matsumoto, Kiiko and Birch, Stephen (1983) *Five Elements and Ten Stems*. Brookline, MA: Paradigm Publications, p.1.

10 Wakefield, Mary Elizabeth (2014) *Constitutional Facial Acupuncture.* London: Churchill Livingstone Elsevier, pp.73–140.

11 TCM is an abbreviation for Traditional Chinese Medicine, which sometimes stipulates different point locations than in Japanese acupuncture treatments. If a point is not specifically designated as being Japanese, you should use the TCM location.

12 Cousto, Hans (2000) *The Cosmic Octave: Origin of Harmony.* Mendocino, CA: Life Rhythm Publications, p.102.

13 See the *Chi-Akra Center for Ageless Aging* website, www.facialacupuncture-wakefieldtechnique.com, for more information about *Facial Soundscapes*™; the training program is comprised of five educational modules that introduce the gamut of Acutonics® tuning forks.

14 Lanzetta, Beverly (2018) *The Monk Within: Embracing a Sacred Way of Life.* Sebastopol, CA: Blue Sapphire Books, p.135.

Chapter 8

1 Preverbal tension manifests as a tightness under the tongue in the anterior digastricus muscle, referred to as the "singer's" muscle. It usually develops prior to the child acquiring verbal skills. This blockage, and the associated tightness, can remain in place for years until released by cranio-sacral treatment in accompaniment with nonverbal sound.

2 Hirschi, Gertrud (2000) *Mudras: Yoga in Your Hands.* San Francisco, CA: Weiser Books, p.2.

3 Larre, Claude, Schatz, Jean, and Rochat de la Valle, Elisabeth (1986) *Survey of Traditional Chinese Medicine.* Columbia, MD: Traditional Acupuncture Institute, pp.213–214.

4 Deadman, Peter, Al-Khafaji, Mazin, and Baker, Kevin (1998) *A Manual of Acupuncture.* London: Journal of Chinese Medicine Publications, p.511.

5 Larre, Schatz, and Rochat de la Valle, *op. cit.*, p.214.

6 Damasio, Antonio (1999) *The Feeling of What Happens.* New York, NY: Harcourt, Brace and Co.

7 Sacks, Oliver (2007) *Musicophilia: Tales of Music and the Brain.* New York, NY: Alfred A. Knopf, p.94.

Chapter 9

1 Cleary, Thomas (translator) (2003) *The Taoist Classics, Volume 4: The Taoist I Ching/I Ching Mandalas.* Boston, MA: Shambhala Publications, p.447.

2 *Ibid.*, p.47.

3 These lines are an indication of damp heat in the Gall Bladder, but are still consistent with a disharmony with the Wood element.

4 Von Bingen, Hildegard (1998) *Physica* (translated by Throop, Priscilla). Rochester, VT: Healing Arts Press, pp.137–156.

5 Strehlow, Wighard, Dr. (2012). *Hildegard of Bingen's Spiritual Remedies* (translated by Strehlow, Karin Anderson). Rochester, VT: Healing Arts Press, p.xiii.

6 Von Bingen, *op. cit.*, p.155.

7 Gienger, Michael (2008) *The Healing Crystal First Aid Manual.* Rochester, VT: Earth Dancer Books.

8 Wakefield, Mary Elizabeth (2014) *Constitutional Facial Acupuncture.* London: Churchill Livingstone Elsevier, pp.323–331.

9 See, for example, Hyde, Lewis (2010) *Trickster Makes This World: Mischief, Myth and Art.* New York, NY: Farrar, Straus and Giroux.

10 Wakefield, *op. cit.*, p.332.

Chapter 10

1 Mary Elizabeth Wakefield.

Bibliography

Abate, Skya Gardner (2001) *The Art of Palpatory Diagnosis in Chinese Medicine.* Edinburgh: Churchill Livingstone.

Apel, Willi (1944) *Harvard Dictionary of Music.* Cambridge, MA: Harvard University Press.

Beaulieu, John (2010) *Human Tuning: Sound Healing with Tuning Forks.* High Falls, NY: Biosonic Enterprises.

Beaulieu, John (2016) *Music and Sound in the Healing Arts: An Energy Approach.* High Falls, NY: Biosonic Enterprises.

Berendt, Joachim-Ernst (1985) *The Third Ear: On Listening to the World.* New York, NY: Henry Holt and Co.

BEC Crew (2016) "Scientists just captured the flash of light that sparks when a sperm meets an egg." Accessed on April 31, 2019 at www.sciencealert.com/scientists-just-captured-the-actual-flash-of-light-that-sparks-when-sperm-meets-an-egg.

Berendt, Joachim-Ernst (1987) *Nada Brahma: The World Is Sound, Music and the Landscape of Consciousness.* New York, NY: Henry Holt and Co.

Brindley, Erica Fox (2012) *Music, Cosmology and the Politics of Harmony in Early China.* Albany, NY: SUNY Press.

Brodie, Renee (1996) *The Healing Tones of Crystal Bowls: Heal Yourself with Sound and Color.* Vancouver, BC: Aroma Art.

Bruyere, Rosalyn L. and Farren, Jeanne (ed.) (1989) *Wheels of Light: A Study of the Chakras, Volume 1.* Sierra Madre, CA: Bon Productions.

Callison, Matt (2007) *Motor Point Index: An Acupuncturist's Guide to Locating and Treating Motor Points.* San Diego, CA: Acu-Sport Seminar Series, LLC.

Campbell, Joseph (1964) *The Masks of God: Occidental Mythology, Volume 3.* New York, NY: Viking Press, pp.21–22.

Carey, Donna and DeMuynck, Marjorie (2002) *There's No Place Like Ohm.* Llano, NM: Devachan Press.

Carey, Donna, Franklin, Ellen, MichelAngelo, Ponton, Judith, and Ponton, Paul (2010) *Acutonics from Galaxies to Cells: Planetary Science, Harmony and Medicine.* Llano, NM: Devachan Press.

Carr, Nicholas (2011) *The Shallows: What the Internet Is Doing to Our Brains.* New York, NY: W. W. Norton & Company.

Chase, Charles and Shima, Miki (2010) *An Exposition on the Eight Extraordinary Vessels: Acupuncture, Alchemy and Herbal Medicine.* Seattle, WA: Eastland Press.

Cleary, Thomas (translator) (2003) *The Taoist Classics, Volume 4: The Taoist I Ching/I Ching Mandalas.* Boston, MA: Shambhala Publications.

Connelly, Diane (1994) *Traditional Acupuncture: The Law of the Five Elements*, 2nd ed. Self-published.

Cousto, Hans (2000) *The Cosmic Octave: Origin of Harmony.* Mendocino, CA: Life Rhythm Publications.

Damasio, Antonio (1999) *The Feeling of What Happens.* New York, NY: Harcourt, Brace and Co.

Deadman, Peter, Al-Khafaji, Mazin, and Baker, Kevin (1998) *A Manual of Acupuncture.* London: Journal of Chinese Medicine Publications.

Dechar, Lori Eve (2006) *Five Spirits: Alchemical Acupuncture for Psychological and Spiritual Healing.* New York, NY: Chiron Publications/Lantern Books.

Denmei, Shudo (2011) *Introduction to Meridian Therapy* (translated by Brown, Stephen). Seattle, WA: Eastland Press.

Ellis, Andrew, Wiseman, Nigel, and Boss, Ken (1989) *Grasping the Wind: An Exploration into the Meaning of Chinese Acupuncture Point Names.* St. Paul, MN: Paradigm Publications.

Ferguson, Kitty (2008) *The Music of Pythagoras: How an Ancient Brotherhood Cracked the Code of the Universe and Lit the Path from Antiquity to Outer Space.* New York, NY: Walker Books.

Fottrell, Quentin (2018) "People spend most of their waking hours staring at screens." Accessed on 21 August, 2019 at https://www.marketwatch.com/story/people-are-spending-most-of-their-waking-hours-staring-at-screens-2018-08-01.

García, Héctor and Miralles, Francesc (2016) *Ikigai: The Japanese Secret to a Long and Happy Life* (translated by Cleary, Heather). New York, NY: Penguin Books.

Gaynor, Mitchell L. (2002) *The Healing Power of Sound: Recovery from Life-Threatening Illness Using Sound, Voice and Music*. Boston, MA: Shambhala Publications.

Gienger, Michael (2008) *The Healing Crystal First Aid Manual*. Rochester, VT: Earthdancer Books.

Gienger, Michael (2009) *Healing Crystals: The A–Z Guide to 430 Gemstones*. Forres: Earthdancer Books.

Gienger, Michael and Goebel, Joachim (2007) *Gem Water: How to Prepare More Than 130 Crystal Waters for Therapeutic Treatments*. Forres: Earthdancer Books.

Gimbutaus, Marija (2001) *The Language of the Goddess*. London: Thames & Hudson.

Gioia, Ted (2006) *Healing Songs*. Durham, NC: Duke University Press.

Golding, Rosin (2008) *The Complete Stems and Branches: Time and Space in Traditional Acupuncture*. London: Churchill Livingstone Elsevier.

Gray, John (1992) *Men Are from Mars, Women Are from Venus: The Classic Guide to Understanding the Opposite Sex*. New York, NY: HarperCollins Publishers.

Gurudas (1989) *Gem Elixirs and Vibrational Healing, Volume 1*. San Rafael, CA: Cassandra Press.

Guthrie, Kenneth Sylvan (translator and compiler) (1988) *The Pythagorean Sourcebook and Library*. Grand Rapids, MI: Phanes Press.

Heline, Corinne (1978) *Healing and Regeneration through Music*. Los Angeles, CA: New Age Press.

Hetherington, Norriss S. (Ed.) (2014) *Encyclopedia of Cosmology (Routledge Revivals): Historical, Philosophical, and Scientific Foundations of Modern Cosmology*. New York, NY: Routledge.

Hirschi, Gertrud (2000) *Mudras: Yoga in Your Hands*. San Francisco, CA: Weiser Books.

Hyde, Lewis (2010) *Trickster Makes This World: Mischief, Myth and Art*. New York, NY: Farrar, Straus and Giroux.

Jacob, Jeffrey H. (2003) *The Acupuncturist's Clinical Handbook*. New York, NY: Integrative Wellness.

James, Jamie (1995) *The Music of the Spheres: Music, Science and the Natural Order of the Universe*. New York, NY: Copernicus Books.

Jansen, Eva Rudy (2002) *Singing Bowls: A Practical Handbook of Instruction and Use*. New Delhi: New Age Books.

Jefferson Lab (n.d.) "Questions and Answers." Accessed on April 25, 2019 at https://education.jlab.org/qa/electron_number.html.

Jespersen, Otto (2016) *Language, Its Nature, Development and Origin*. Palala Press.

Jung, Carl (1962) *Memories, Dreams, Reflections*. New York, NY: Pantheon Books.

Kaptchuk, Ted (1983) *The Web That Has No Weaver: Understanding Chinese Medicine*. Chicago, IL: Congdon & Weed.

Keown, Daniel (2014) *The Spark in the Machine: How the Science of Acupuncture Explains the Mysteries of Western Medicine*. London: Singing Dragon.

Kerenyi, Carl (1951) *The Gods of the Greeks*. London: Thames & Hudson, p.18.

Khan, Hazrat Inayat (1983) *The Music of Life*. New Lebanon, NY: Omega Press.

Koestler, Arthur (2017) *The Sleepwalkers: A History of Man's Changing View of the Universe*. London: Penguin Arkana.

Koren, Leonard (2008) *Wabi-Sabi for Artists, Designers, Poets and Philosophers*. Point Reyes, CA: Imperfect Press.

Lanzetta, Beverly (2018) *The Monk Within: Embracing a Sacred Way of Life*. Sebastopol, CA: Blue Sapphire Books.

Larre, Claude, Schatz, Jean, and Rochat de la Valle, Elisabeth (1986) *Survey of Traditional Chinese Medicine*. Columbia, MD: Traditional Acupuncture Institute.

Levitin, Daniel (2006) *This Is Your Brain on Music: The Science of a Human Obsession*. New York, NY: Dutton Adult.

Levitin, Daniel (2008) *The World in Six Songs: How the Musical Brain Created Human Nature*. New York, NY: Dutton (Penguin).

MacKenzie, Janice (2002) *Discovering the Five Elements One Day at a Time*. New Hope, PA: Wind Palace Publishing.

Mains, Richard and Eipper, Betty A. (1999) *The Neuropeptides*. Philadelphia, PA: Lippincott-Raven.

Mannes, Elena (2011) *The Power of Music: Pioneering Discoveries in the New Science of Song*. New York, NY: Walker & Company.

Matsumoto, Kiiko and Birch, Stephen (1983) *Five Elements and Ten Stems: Nan Ching Theory, Diagnostics and Practice*. Brookline, MA: Paradigm Publications.

Matsumoto, Kiiko and Birch, Stephen (1988) *Hara Diagnosis: Reflections on the Sea*. Brookline, MA: Paradigm Publications.

McTaggart, Lynne (2007) *The Intention Experiment: Using Your Thoughts to Change Your Life and the World*. New York, NY: Free Press.

Meyer, Kathi (1952) "The Eight Gregorian Modes on the Cluny Capitals." *Art Bulletin 34*, 2, 75–94.

Mithen, Steven (2007) *The Singing Neanderthals: The Origins of Music, Language, Mind and Body.* Cambridge, MA: Harvard University Press.

Ni, Yitian (1996) *Navigating the Channels of Traditional Chinese Medicine.* San Diego, CA: Oriental Medical Center.

OUP (2013) *Oxford English Dictionary* (11th edition). Oxford: Oxford University Press.

Perret, Daniel (2005) *Sound Healing with the Five Elements: Sound Instruments Sound Therapy Sound Energy.* Havelte: Binkey Kok Publications.

Perry, Frank (2014) *Himalayan Sound Revelations: The Complete Singing Bowl Book.* London: Polair Publishing.

Rudhyar, Dane (1982) *The Magic of Tone and the Art of Music.* Boston, MA: Shambhala Books.

Sacks, Oliver (2007) *Musicophilia: Tales of Music and the Brain.* New York, NY: Alfred A. Knopf.

Schneider, Achim (2014) "Ice-age musicians fashioned ivory flute." Accessed on April 24, 2019 at www.nature.com/news/2004/041213/full/041213-14.html.

Shea, Peter (2015) *Alchemy of the Extraordinary: A Journey into the Heart of the Meridian Matrix.* Asheville, NC: Self-published.

Shlain, Leonard (2004) *Sex, Time and Power: How Women's Sexuality Shaped Human Evolution.* New York, NY: Penguin Books.

Sigerson, John and Wolfe, Kathy (1992) *A Manual on the Rudiments of Tuning and Registration. Book 1: Introduction and Human Singing Voice.* Washington, DC: Schiller Institute (Kindle version).

Sjöö, Monica and Mor, Barbara (1991) *The Great Cosmic Mother: Rediscovering the Religion of the Earth.* San Francisco, CA: Harper San Francisco.

Strehlow, Wighard (2002) *Hildegard of Bingen's Spiritual Remedies* (translated by Strehlow, Karin Anderson). Rochester, VT: Healing Arts Press.

Strehlow, Wighard and Hertkz, Gottfried (1988) *Hildegard of Bingen's Medicine* (translated by Strehlow, Karin Anderson). Santa Fe, NM: Bear & Company.

Tame, David (1984) *The Secret Power of Music: The Transformation of Self and Society through Musical Energy.* Rochester, VT: Destiny Books.

Taylor, T. (translator) (1818) *Iamblichus' Life of Pythagoras or Pythagoric Life.* London: J.M. Watkins.

Tomatis, Alfred A. (1991) *The Conscious Ear.* Barrytown, NY: Station Hill Press.

Travell, Janet G. and Simons, David G. (1983) *Myofascial Pain and Dysfunction: The Trigger Point Manual,* Volumes 1 and 2. Baltimore, MD: Williams and Wilkins.

Tsay, Chia-Jung (2013) "Sight over sound in the judgment of music performance." *Proceedings of the National Academy of Sciences 110,* 36, 14580–14585.

Twicken, David (2013) *Eight Extraordinary Channels: Qi Jing Ba Mai, A Handbook for Clinical Practice and Nei Dan Inner Meditation.* London: Singing Dragon.

University of Washington (2001) "Brains of Deaf People Rewire to 'Hear' Music." *ScienceDaily.* Accessed on April 29, 2019 at www.sciencedaily.com/releases/2001/11/011128035455.htm.

Unschuld, Paul U. (1985) *Medicine in China: A History of Ideas.* Berkeley and Los Angeles, CA: University of California Press.

Von Bingen, Hildegard (1998) *Physica* (translated by Throop, Priscilla). Rochester, VT: Healing Arts Press.

Voss, Angela (n.d.) *The Music of the Spheres: Ficino and Renaissance Harmonia.* Accessed on April 29, 2019 at http://gnosticacademy.com/voss-a-the-music-of-the-spheres-ficino-and-renaissance-harmonia.

Voss, Angela (n.d.) *The Theurgic Symbol: Musico-Magic Therapeutics in the Sixteenth Century,* p.1. Accessed on April 30, 2019 at www.academia.edu/32728827/Music_and_Magic.

Wakefield, Mary Elizabeth (2014) *Constitutional Facial Acupuncture.* London: Churchill Livingstone Elsevier.

Walker, Barbara (1983) *The Woman's Encyclopedia of Myths and Secrets.* New York, NY: HarperCollins Publishers.

Wallnöfer, Heinrich and von Rottauscher, Anna (1965) *Chinese Folk Medicine and Acupuncture.* New York, NY: Bell Publishing Company.

Wells, Jain (2018) *Gong Consciousness: Self-Healing through the Power of Sound.* Choiceless Awareness Communications.

Wu, Wei-P'ing (1962) *Chinese Acupuncture* (translated by Lavier, Jacques). Whitstable: Straker Brothers.

Wu, Zhongxian and Wu, Karin Taylor (2014) *Heavenly Stems and Earthly Branches—TianGan DiZhi: The Heat of Chinese Wisdom Traditions.* London: Singing Dragon.

About the Authors

Mary Elizabeth Wakefield L.Ac. M.S. M.M. ───────────

Mary Elizabeth Wakefield, the internationally recognized author of the book *Constitutional Facial Acupuncture*, is an acclaimed teacher, an acupuncturist, herbalist, Acutonics® and Zen Shiatsu practitioner, cranio-sacral therapist, and a professional opera singer. Acknowledged to be a leading international authority on facial acupuncture, with 30-plus years of clinical professional experience as a healing practitioner, she has personally trained close to 5500 healthcare practitioners from five continents in her treatment protocols.

She maintains a private practice on the Upper East Side of Manhattan, in New York City.

MichelAngelo M.F.A. C.T.M. ───────────────

An opera singer, classical composer, pianist, medical astrologer, healer, diviner, and writer, MichelAngelo served as Advisor, Astrological Medicine and Musical Studies to Acutonics® Institute of Integrative Medicine, LLC, and is a co-author of the textbook, *Acutonics from Galaxies to Cells: Planetary Science, Harmony and Medicine.* He has written several articles on medical astrology for *Oriental Medicine Journal.* Other articles have appeared in *Dell Horoscope* and *Infinity Astrological Journal.*

MichelAngelo recently self-published an e-book of original essays, *Random Ramblings of an Astrological Autodidact,* available on Amazon.

Index